99 Prompts

to

Mindfulness

and

Well-Being

A journal to help you discover
self-awareness through mindful
practices and help improve your
overall well-being

Ricki Wax

Published by Ricki Wax

Book Design by Kory Kirby
KORYKIRBY.COM

ISBN: 978-1-7358305-0-6 (hardback)
ISBN: 978-1-7358305-1-3 (paperback)

Printed in the United States of America

For my family.
I love you all and appreciate your support.

Contents

These first set of prompts will set a foundation to establishing a mind-fulness and well-being journey. We'll explore topics such as defining what mindfulness is — a variety of exercises, techniques, and methods to which you can always come back. I like to think of this section as learning the basics.

In this next section, we'll start to explore self-awareness. At the end of these sets of prompts, I want you to come to the realization of who you are and accept that you are enough. Many prompts will involve self-affir-mation, self-love, self-care. Take your time going through these prompts to ensure you're doing the work.

In this next section, we'll explore emotions and senses. The idea of being present is understanding how your body reacts in certain situa-tions. These prompts will have you step outside your comfort zone and be uncomfortable. Linger in the discomfort and explore the different emotions from the various prompts.

Transformation

Be the change you want to see! These next few prompts will focus on areas of growth and maturation. We'll explore prompts related to your current events and future goals. In order to achieve transformation and triumph you must first explore what makes you well.

Inspiration

As we round out our last section of our journal. I wanted to end on a high note of inspirational prompts. These prompts will explore your purpose and passion. I've designed them to invoke excitement in your future. A key piece of advice as you explore this section is to ask yourself, do I need to wait for one day or can I make this day one?

Journaling

Here are a few additional pages for you to expand on prompts you've really enjoyed or take some additional time to reflect on the better version of you!

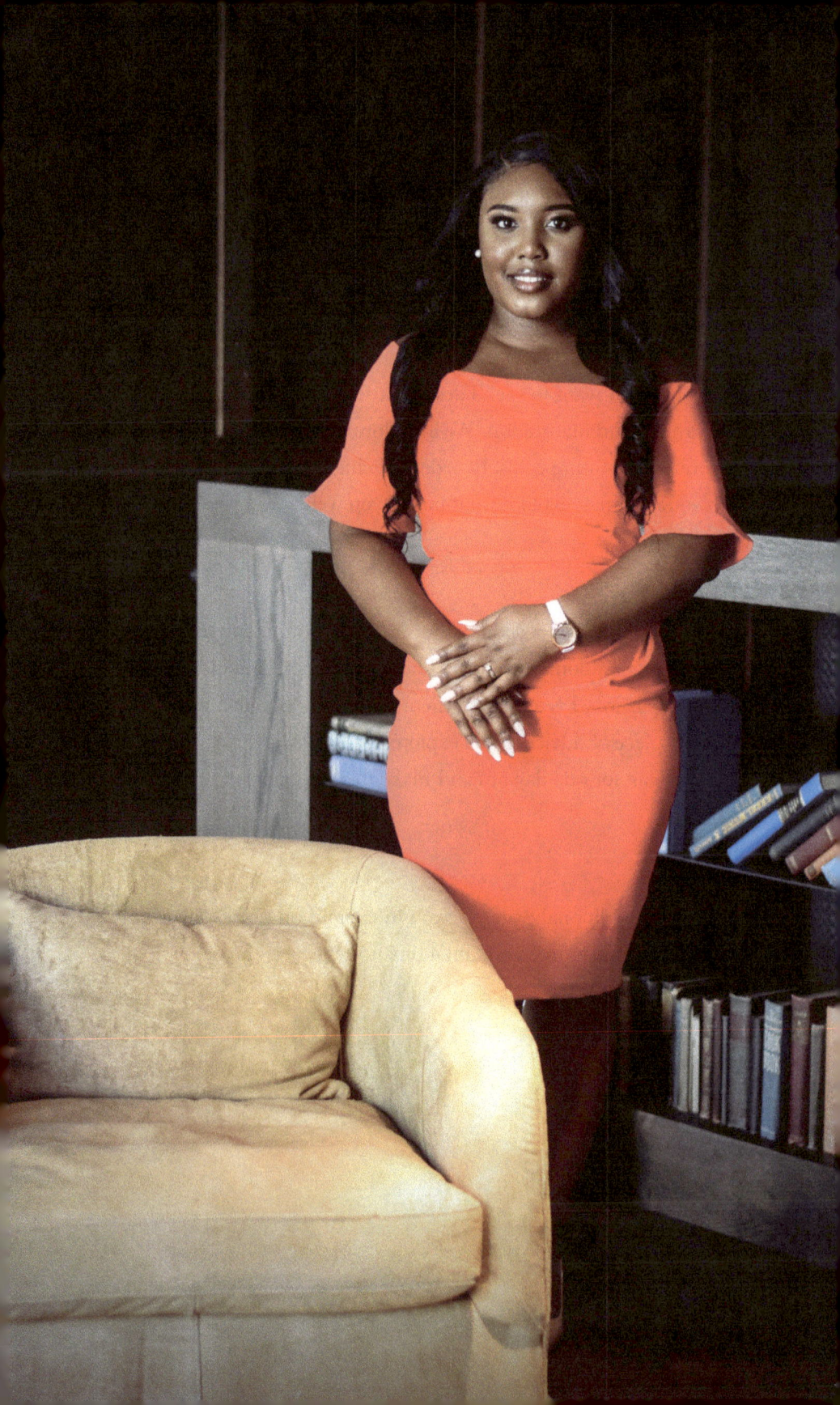

A letter from the author

*I*STARTED WRITING THESE JOURNAL PROMPTS AFTER taking a course that encouraged me to open up and search deep inside myself. Over the last year, I have felt like I was existing more than really living, which is why I was excited to take this training. My eyes were opened as we went through various stages of how my overall mindfulness and self-aware-ness affects total performance. Not just in my work, but in my everyday life. I knew then that I had to make a change — a change to be better. I wanted to live my life out loud. Be Bold. Be Proud. Live Out Loud. I wanted to be intentional in my actions and behaviors. I wanted the universe to appreciate the gifts I had to offer and definitely take advantage of all life's gems. I've learned to take both the good and the bad that life throws at you. You see, for every failure, there is a lesson. For every joy, there is sorrow. And that, my friend, is how you learn to appreciate both the wins and the losses of life. Each day, I wake up with breath in my lungs, I thank a Higher power for allowing me to be mindful of the wind beneath my wings, the blood that flows through my veins, the energy that sends shockwaves through my soul, and the earth that rumbles below my feet.

May this journal be the tool which sets you on fire. Use it to get you started on your journey to mindfulness and well-being. Live a life you love, and don't let anyone stop you!

Education

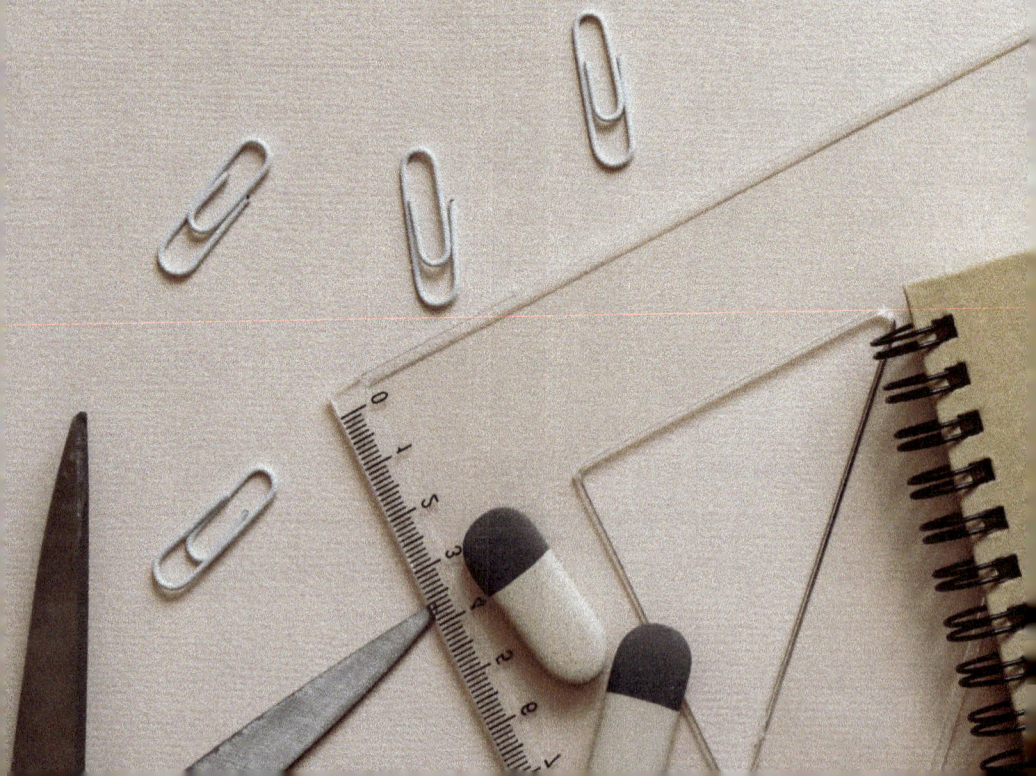

These first set of prompts will set a foundation to establishing a mindfulness and well-being journey. We'll explore topics such as defining what mindfulness is — a variety of exercises, techniques, and methods to which you can always come back. I like to think of this section as learning the basics.

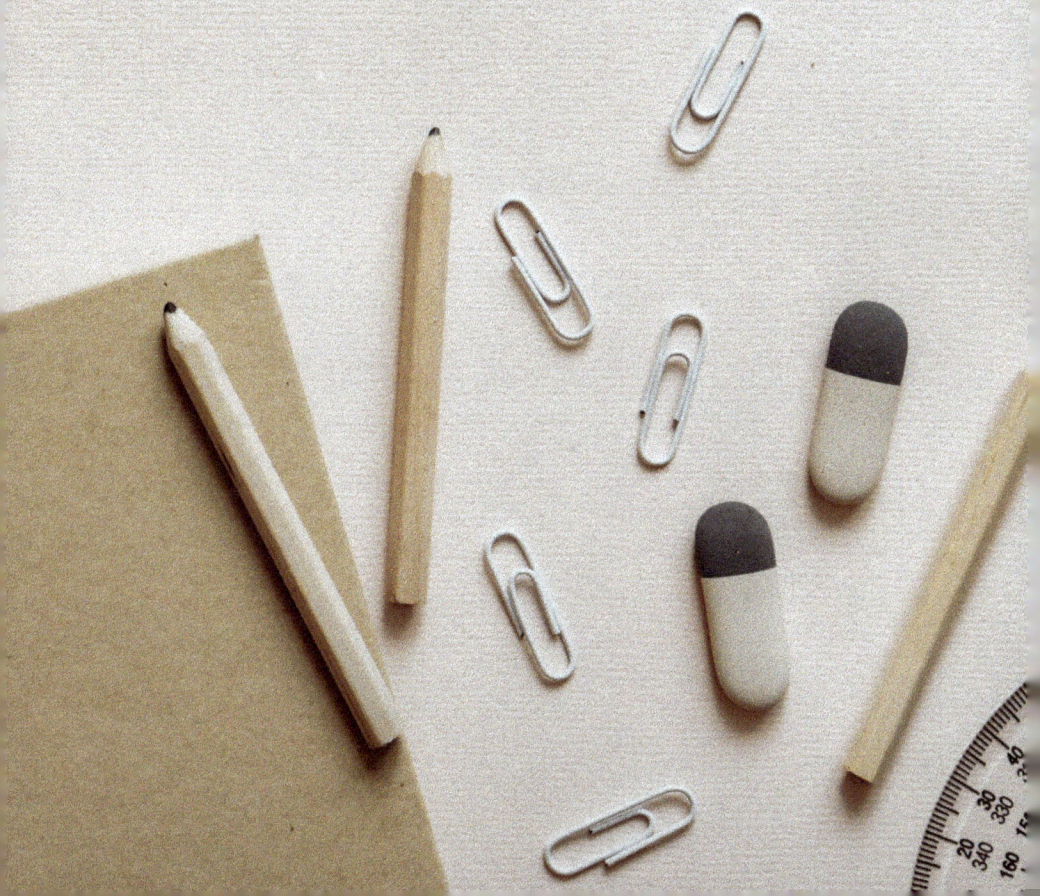

1

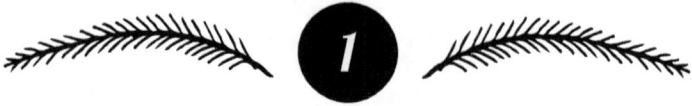

"Mindfulness means paying attention to what's happening in the present moment in the mind, body, and external environment with an attitude of curiosity and kindness. Mindfulness is a way of being in a wise and purposeful relationship with one's experience, both inwardly and outwardly" (Mindful Nation UK Report). Take a moment and close your eyes. Silence your thoughts. Be present in this moment. Breathe and count backwards from 10. Reflect on what comes up for you. Live in the moment.

....

....

....

....

....

....

....

....

....

....

....

....

....

....

2

Mindfulness improves physical health. I started my wellness journey earlier this year after seeing Oprah's Vision 2020 Tour. At the time, I never considered myself a runner or "in shape" athlete. Slowly, I began to take 20-minute. walks around the neighborhood. I even downloaded the C25k app to help track my progress. My 20-minute walks then turned into 30 minutes. A slight jog, and eventually I was able to do a few laps. I began to have more energy and even feel better about my health in general. I'd like to encourage you to try one physical activity today. It can be a walk, a dance around the living room, a play date with your children. Full creative license. What was your exercise? How did you feel while doing it? What kept you focused?

....

....

....

....

....

....

....

....

....

....

....

....

3

Mindfulness improves mental health. According to a study done by mentalhealth.org, evidence suggests by becoming more self-aware — being able to manage your thoughts through breathing and meditation — has led to improvements in mental health. Let's practice a deep breathing exercise. Stretch out your hands. Allow your thoughts to wander during this exercise. Focus on your breath. Get distracted. Welcome the distraction, and then let it go and re-focus on your breath. Go as long as you need to. Afterwards, journal what came up for you during this exercise.

....

....

....

....

....

....

....

....

....

....

....

....

....

....

4

Mindful eating is the practice of intentionally slowing down to savor each flavorful bite of food. For at least one meal today, try mindful eating. What did you discover? How was your meal? What did you feel while doing this?

....

....

....

....

....

....

....

....

....

....

....

....

....

....

....

....

....

....

5

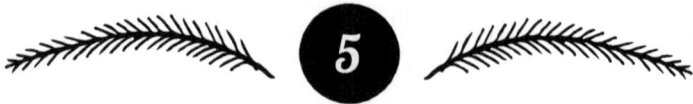

Practice mindful meditation for one minute. Set a timer for one minute. Focus on your breathing. If your mind starts to wander, allow the distractions to come in. Welcome them. Acknowledge them. Then go back to your breathing. Try not to have any resistance. Now write about your exercise. Were you able to focus? Where did your mind go?

....

....

....

....

....

....

....

....

....

....

....

....

....

....

....

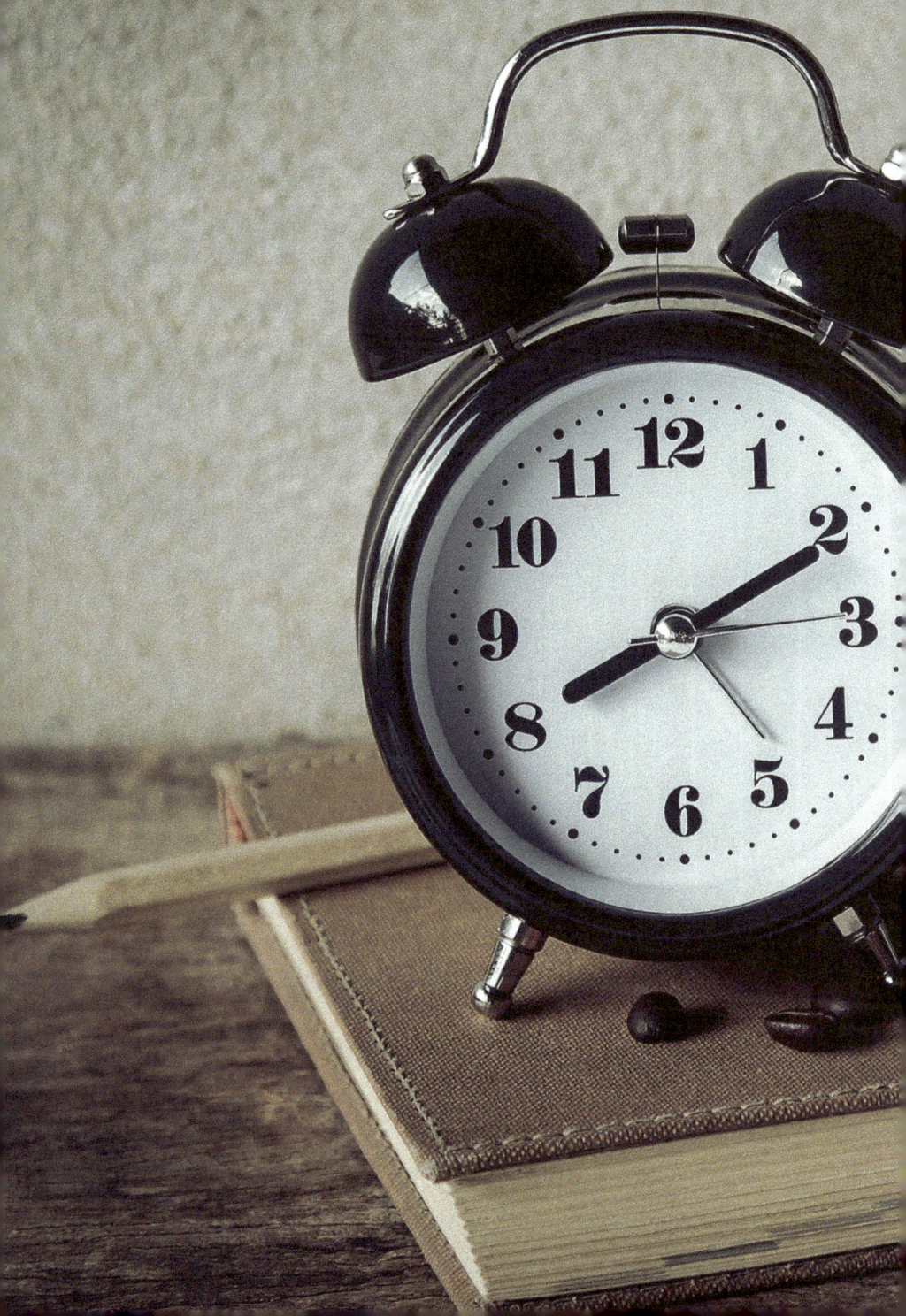

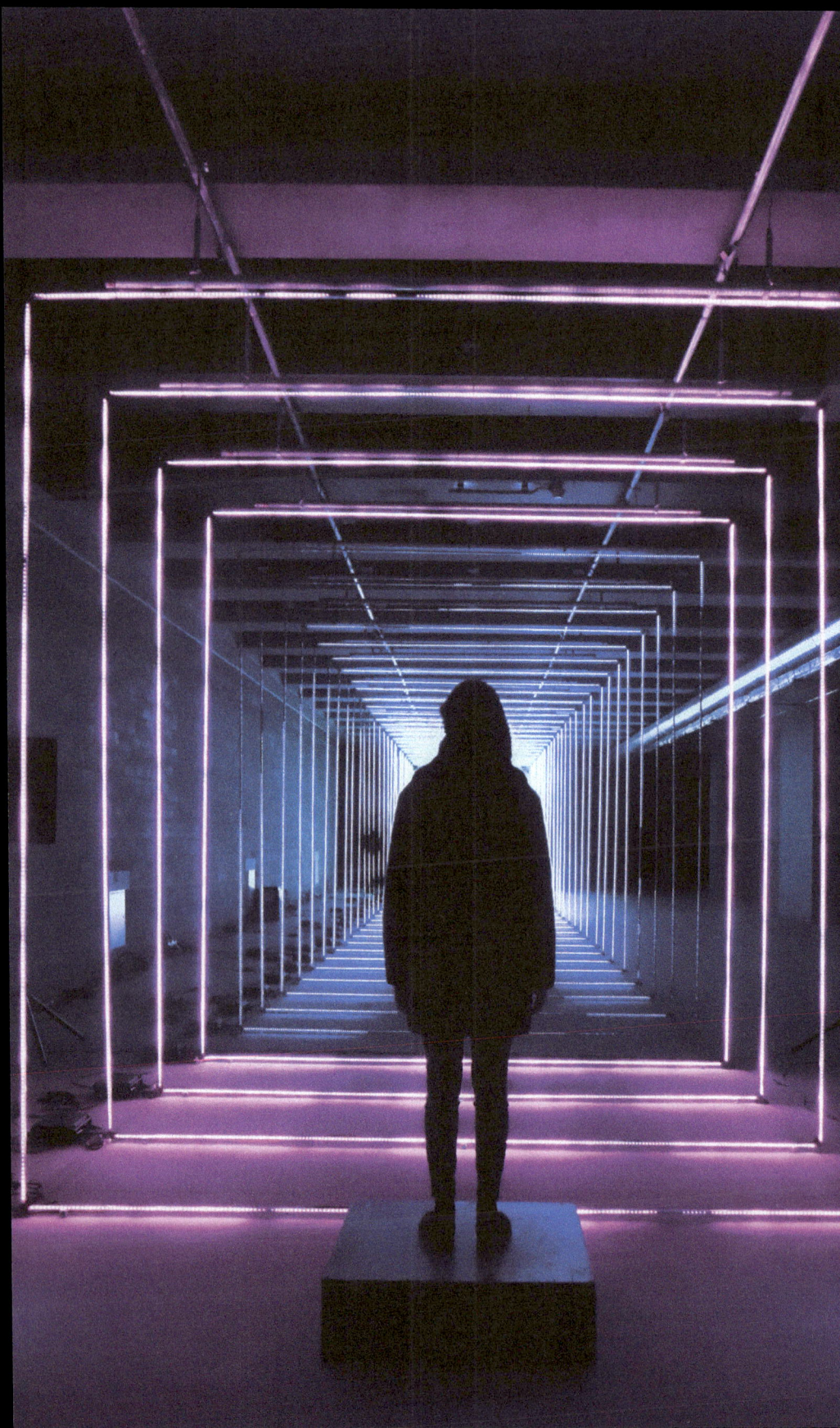

6

Body Scan Mindfulness is an exercise which allows you to take notice of your body. Get into a comfortable position and start to scan your body from head to toe. Start from your feet, moving slowly towards your toes, up to your ankles, and continue on until you reach the tip of your nose, onwards to the top of your head. Be sure to take at least 10- 15 minute. with this exercise as it allows you to feel any tension throughout your body. How hard was it to focus? What elements of your body did you feel while doing the exercise?

....

....

....

....

....

....

....

....

....

....

....

....

....

....

7

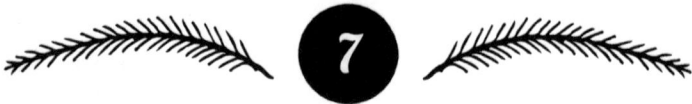

Loving Kindness Meditation (LKM) is a popular self-care technique used to boost well-being and reduce stress. According to a study by mental health resource website Verywell Mind, this practice allows for forgiveness, self-love, connection to others, and self-acceptance. For one minute, practice "May I be happy, may I be safe, may I be kind, may I be love, may I be healthy, and may I give and receive appreciation today." As you enjoy these moments of joy and happiness, start to reflect these same feelings towards someone close to you. "May __ be happy, may __be safe, may __ be kind, may __ be love." And so on. If you are mentally in control, extend those same emotions to strangers in the universe. "May they be happy. May they be safe. May they be kind." And so on. Reflect on this exercise, and see what comes up.

....

....

....

....

....

....

....

....

....

....

....

....

8

Cultivating gratitude through senses builds mindfulness. In this exercise, we will use a moment of meditation to clear any dark thoughts and tune your awareness to focus on life's little delights. *Start with deep breaths. Bring your mind to a sight you are grateful for. Bring your nose to a scent you appreciate. Wiggle your fingers to touch and feel the blood in your veins. Position your heart to gently receive this moment of appreciation for the space you are in. Look around and revel in the greatness of your appreciation. Reflect on this exercise.*

....
....
....
....
....
....
....
....
....
....
....
....
....
....
....

9

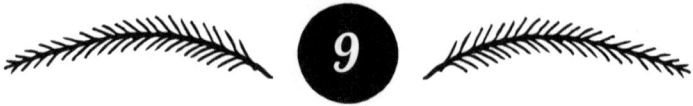

According to an article in Forbes, sunlight exposure causes a rise in serotonin levels.1 This is also known as the "happiness" hormone. Sunshine has been linked to improved mood, decreased depression, and manageable anxiety. I believe this is one of the reasons I enjoy being outside so much — feeling the rays brush my face gives me energy. *For today's prompt, imagine you are outside, or if you can, go outside. Spend a day in the sun and reflect on what mood you're feeling. Close your eyes and focus on the bright, sunny skies. What comes up for you?*

....

....

....

....

....

....

....

....

....

....

....

....

....

....

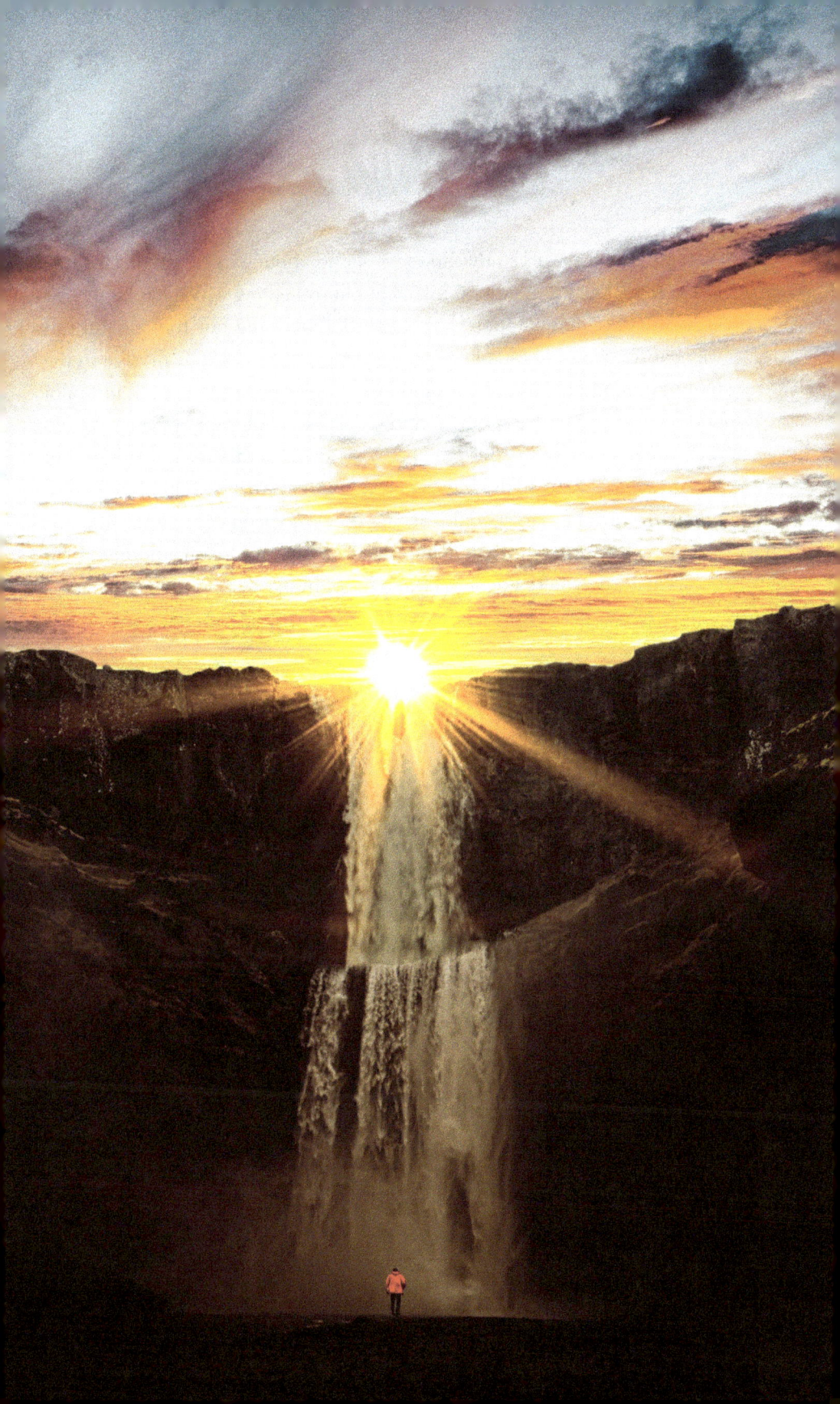

10

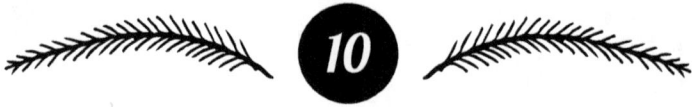

Autopilot: A Harvard study shows we spend about 47 percent of our time lost in our thoughts—either thinking about something which has happened in the past or may happen in the future. Operating our thoughts in this way causes us to run on autopilot, meaning we are not fully present in the moment. The purpose of mindfulness is to be present. Get off autopilot and be present. Take a moment and reflect on all of your activities you do on autopilot. For some, this may be work, gym, dinner for the kiddos, but for others, this may be driving the same route to work or school every day, or eating with the same people. Seeing the same people for happy hour, or tea, or coffee. Write down activities during which you're on autopilot, then describe a way you're going to switch it up this week.

....

....

....

....

....

....

....

....

....

....

....

Mindful Listening: engage with someone and have a mindful conversation. In order to do this, practice the 3 A's. Attention, Attitude, and Adjustment. When focused, you are paying attention in that present moment of what the other person is saying. You have pushed your own thoughts, anxieties, and worries aside to really hear what the other person is saying. Attitude is having the right attitude when listening; simply put, you have an open mind and curious heart. You welcome what the other person may be feeling when speaking. Lastly, adjustment is positioning yourself to adjust to the story the other person is telling, allowing them to reach a point of climax in their story. This could be them needing advice, releasing tension, or sharing wonderful news. Be prepared to adjust your position and refrain from interrupting or jumping to any conclusions before they finish the conversation. Practice having a mindful listening session with someone, and then come back and reflect on this prompt.

....

....

....

....

....

....

....

....

....

....

What's something you're often misunderstood about?

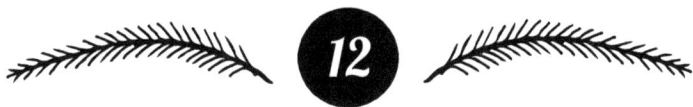

Mindful conversation is the art of being fully present, open, honest, curious, and relating to someone with compassion. Mindful conversation happens once you master mindful listening. I often joke with people about "surface talk." I have a friend who has a shirt which says, "I hate small talk," and I always laugh at that shirt. You see, small talk is nice in the appropriate areas, but I enjoy getting to know people for who they are. I enjoy peeling back the different layers. I guess that's why I went into human resources. I've also been told it was a gift because people feel comfortable sharing with me. I encourage you to go out and have a mindful conversation with someone you know or someone you'd like to know more about. It's those moments which make us all human and spreads a little more love and compassion in the world. Come back and reflect on why you chose that person, how the conversation went, and what you'd like to know next time. Don't have any conversation starters? Here's a few: What are you most passionate about? What's your favorite movie, and why? Who inspires you? What's something you're often misunderstood about?

....

....

....

....

....

....

....

....

....

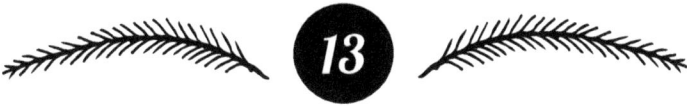

Shift your mindset. Martin Seligman is known as the father of positive psychology. *"Positive psychology is the scientific study of what makes life most worth living" (Peterson, 2008).* Seligman teaches optimistic thinking vs. pessimistic logic. Positive psychology focuses on our strengths instead of weaknesses. This science focuses on compassion, gratitude, life worth living, and resilience. Reflect on your most recent let-down. Are you thinking positively or negatively? Describe your experience in your journal today, and focus on the silver lining from that experience.

....

....

....

....

....

....

....

....

....

....

....

....

....

....

14

Remember, mindfulness is all about the ability to train the mind, allow for self-compassion, reflection, change, and the flexibility between different methods and exercises. I want to introduce you to the three-minute breathing space. This technique is broken down into three sections. One per minute. *In the first minute: answer the question, "How am I doing right now?" Focus only on feelings, thoughts, and sensations that come up for you. The second minute is spent focusing your mind only on your breath. Inhale and Exhale. Feel the air on your skin. Observe your chest rise and fall. The last minute is for moving your attention to how your body responds to your breathing. Focus on multiple parts of your body. What are your hands doing? Is the air hot or cold? Did you get goosebumps? Reflect and write about this exercise.*

....

....

....

....

....

....

....

....

....

....

....

....

Realization

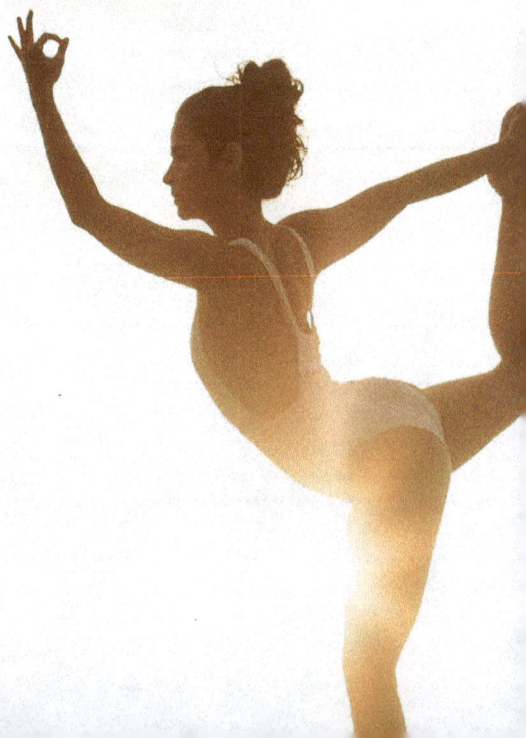

In this next section, we'll start to explore self-awareness. At the end of these sets of prompts, I want you to come to the realization of who you are and accept that you are enough. Many prompts will involve self-affirmation, self-love, self-care. Take your time going through these prompts to ensure you're doing the work.

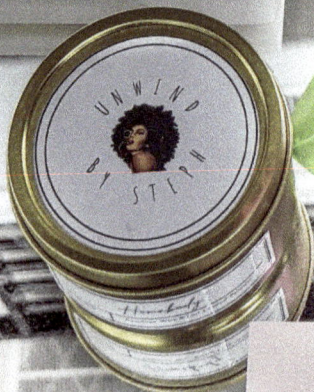

15

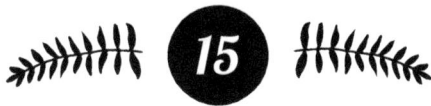

Self-affirmation is a form of self-love. Write down at least 10 self-affirming statements about yourself. For example: "I am enough. I am talented and gifted. I have what it takes to be successful. I am loved." Now you try.

....

....

....

....

....

....

....

....

....

....

....

....

....

....

....

....

....

16

What are some of your greatest strengths? What comes to mind immediately? Are you a connector? Are you a math genius? Are you physically fit? Do you have the ability to see the bigger picture? Perhaps you're good with people? Just start writing.

....

....

....

....

....

....

....

....

....

....

....

....

....

....

....

....

17

In this exercise, I want you to reach out to 2-3 friends, and ask them what they would say your greatest strengths are. What are the characteristics and traits they see in you? Now reflect on each of these, and see if they're connected to how you perceive yourself.

....

....

....

....

....

....

....

....

....

....

....

....

....

....

....

....

....

18

Victor Strecher at the University of Michigan in Ann Arbor, author of the book *Life on Purpose*, suggests identifying different values and goals for four domains of your life: family, work, community, and personal growth according to an article by New Scientist.[2] Take a moment to journal about each of these areas and the legacy you'd like to leave behind for each of them.

....

....

....

....

....

....

....

....

....

....

....

....

....

....

....

....

19

Life is best lived one day at a time, one step at a time. Write down one thing you'd like to accomplish today. Focus on just one goal in order to avoid overwhelming yourself. Now, take a moment and practice mindful walking. Consider taking a slow or moderate walk for five minutes, and ask yourself: why is this the one thing you'd like to accomplish? What level of satisfaction would it provide for you?

....

....

....

....

....

....

....

....

....

....

....

....

....

....

20

Carpe Diem! Seize the day. Let's jump into how you want to seize the day today. Write a list of things you want to accomplish today. As someone who enjoys to-do lists, I often find satisfaction in crossing things off my list once I've completed them. I'd like for you to try this; it can be something you want to do today, or a list for the week. Here are some suggestions: 1. Fold my laundry. 2. Update my resume. 3. Reach out to my parents. 4. Check on a friend. What are some things you'd like to accomplish today?

21

Hyperconnectivity and overstimulation through social media have taken over this generation. Let's try slowing things down. Imagine a simpler life. What are the basic necessities you'd need? How would you live? Describe your fundamentals.

....

....

....

....

....

....

....

....

....

....

....

....

....

....

....

....

....

....

22

The best part of mindful meditation is the work you do on the inside is reflected on the outside. This will allow you to form deeper relationships both professionally and personally. Today, let's reflect inward. What is inside your heart, mind, body, and soul that you'd like to work on?

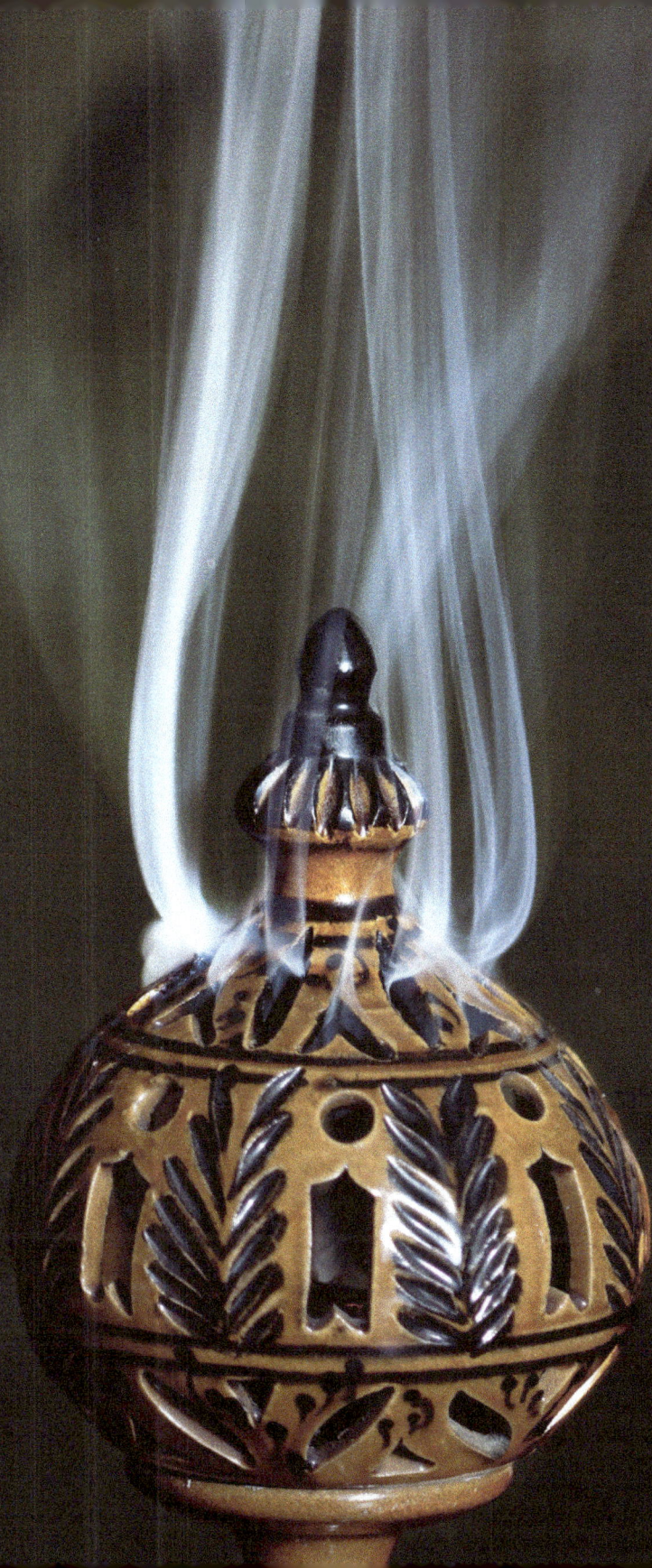

23

A 1999 study linked journaling to reducing stress and anxiety in a medical situation.[3] In 1999, Joshua Smyth and Arthur Stone and colleagues at SUNY at Stony Brook assigned patients with asthma and rheumatoid arthritis either to write about the most stressful event of their lives or to write about a neutral topic. Four months later, asthma patients in the experimental group showed improvements in lung function and arthritis patients in the experimental group showed a reduction in disease severity. In all, 47 percent of the patients who went through stressful events showed relevant improvement, whereas only 24 percent of the control group showed mild improvement. How has mindful meditations and self-awareness exercises from this journal helped you so far?

....

....

....

....

....

....

....

....

....

....

....

24

Honesty is the best policy. Sometimes we aren't completely honest with ourselves. It all starts here. What are some things you're holding back? If you want to live an honest life with others, you must first start being honest with yourself.

....

....

....

....

....

....

....

....

....

....

....

....

....

....

....

....

25

"Leadership is the ability to serve others" (Ricki Wax). It took me a while to figure out the way I wanted to show up as a leader. What way did I want to measure my success? Over the past year, I realized my leadership style and the way I connect with others works uniquely for me. I encourage you to take a moment and self-reflect on your leadership style. What is your perception of an outstanding leader and how are you measuring up?

....
....
....
....
....
....
....
....
....
....
....
....
....
....
....

26

"Before you are a leader, success is all about growing yourself. When you become a leader, success is all about growing others" (Jack Welch). Self-awareness and self-management are all about how you want to show up for others around you. It's essential you put yourself together first before helping others. Are you self-aware? Reflect.

....

....

....

....

....

....

....

....

....

....

....

....

....

....

....

27

Vulnerability can be your greatest strength. Breathe and be vulnerable. People want to see that you're human and you have feelings. Over the course of this journey, I've noticed that striving for perfection actually gets me less results than owning up to my flaws and imperfections. One of the reasons I love the people I love is because they love that I'm perfectly imperfect. They accept me for who I am, and that's okay with me. How do you show your vulnerability?

....

....

....

....

....

....

....

....

....

....

....

....

....

....

28

"Once I became friends with my anxiety, that's when I started setting boundaries in our relationship" (Ricki Wax). I've always suffered from overthinking, being overly anxious on what's to come or what has passed, and I never really knew how to interpret this until a couple of years ago when I started going to therapy. It was then that someone was finally able to put into words all the emotions I'd been feeling since I was younger. You see, I'd always been captain of my cheerleading team, or all-district in my high school—I even won a few superlatives and college accolades. In all these things, I always felt that was just what was expected of me. The "freak out" in my mind was normal, whether I won or didn't win. I transitioned to the real world, got some real medical benefits, and actually started to take advantage of what I'd been blessed with. It's easier to have the resources and not use them than to not have them and complain. I'm glad I did, and now I've been able to manage my anxiety a lot better. You see, my anxiety fuels me to have healthy stress. I know what you're thinking: "healthy stress." The easiest way to define this is when I have a tight deadline, or a project to complete, and I hear it cheering me on because I've come out on top time and time again. You feel relieved and sometimes euphoric because you made it through! But I also know when my stress and anxiety weighs me down or holds me back with circumstances I can't change. That's when I have to understand, now is not the time nor the place to allow negative thoughts to occupy my mind nor body. It's through these healthy boundaries I've been able to cultivate a relationship with my anxiety and healthy stress. I encourage you, if you suffer from anxiety, depression, people-pleasing, or getting lost in your thoughts, brainstorm some ways you can set boundaries with your mental health.

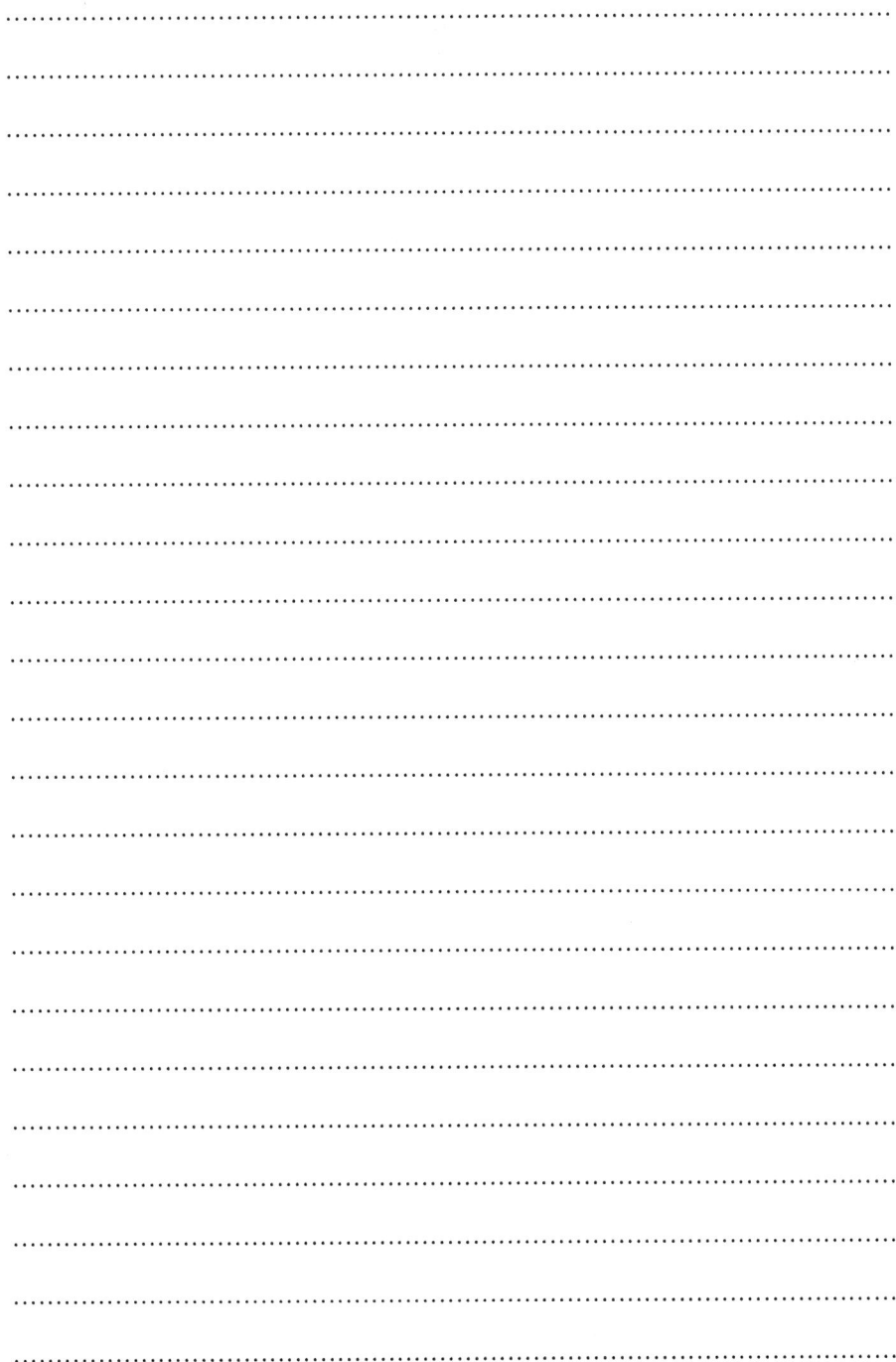

"You can't have self-love without having self-care" (Ricki Wax). If you love yourself, then you'll care about what you eat, what you do, and how you treat yourself. Take a moment to take yourself on a date. Write down all the places you'll go. Describe them in detail—the food you'll eat, the smells you'll smell, and the atmosphere around.

··

··

··

··

··

··

··

··

··

··

··

··

··

··

I read a quote which says, "Choosing to love myself is where I find my power"(Alex Elle). This resonates so much with me in this state of mindfulness and being fully present. There's always going to be this nagging voice which tries to tell you that you aren't good enough, or not pushing hard enough or that you need more despite where you are in. Say hello to this. Welcome this voice and then tell them to **KICK ROCKS!** Because if you choose to love yourself, regardless of where you are, this is truly where you find your power. This is where you rise to any occasion and you own that moment. Own your greatness! Let's try an acceptance exercise. *You can light a candle, or choose a photo and stare at it. Focus your attention in the same spot and start saying all of the things you love about yourself. Reflect once you've finished.* What came up for you during this time?

....

....

....

....

....

....

....

....

....

....

31

"You must love and care for yourself, because that's when the best comes out" (Tina Turner). As a motivational speaker, I always encourage people to put on their own oxygen masks before helping someone else. I need to be okay so that I can be a better shoulder for you to lean on. What are some ways you practice self-care? How are you ensuring you're the best version of yourself to present to the outside world? I like to indulge in massage therapy, counseling, and dance. It's very soothing to reconnect with me, Ricki.

You have to invest in yourself before you can invest in someone else. You must be able to bring your whole self into a relationship. Forget the idea that you are meant to complete someone; rather, let them enhance you, because relationships are all about building together. Take a moment and write down a relationship you'd like to invest in. What tangible steps will you take today to invest?

....

....

....

....

....

....

....

....

....

....

....

....

....

....

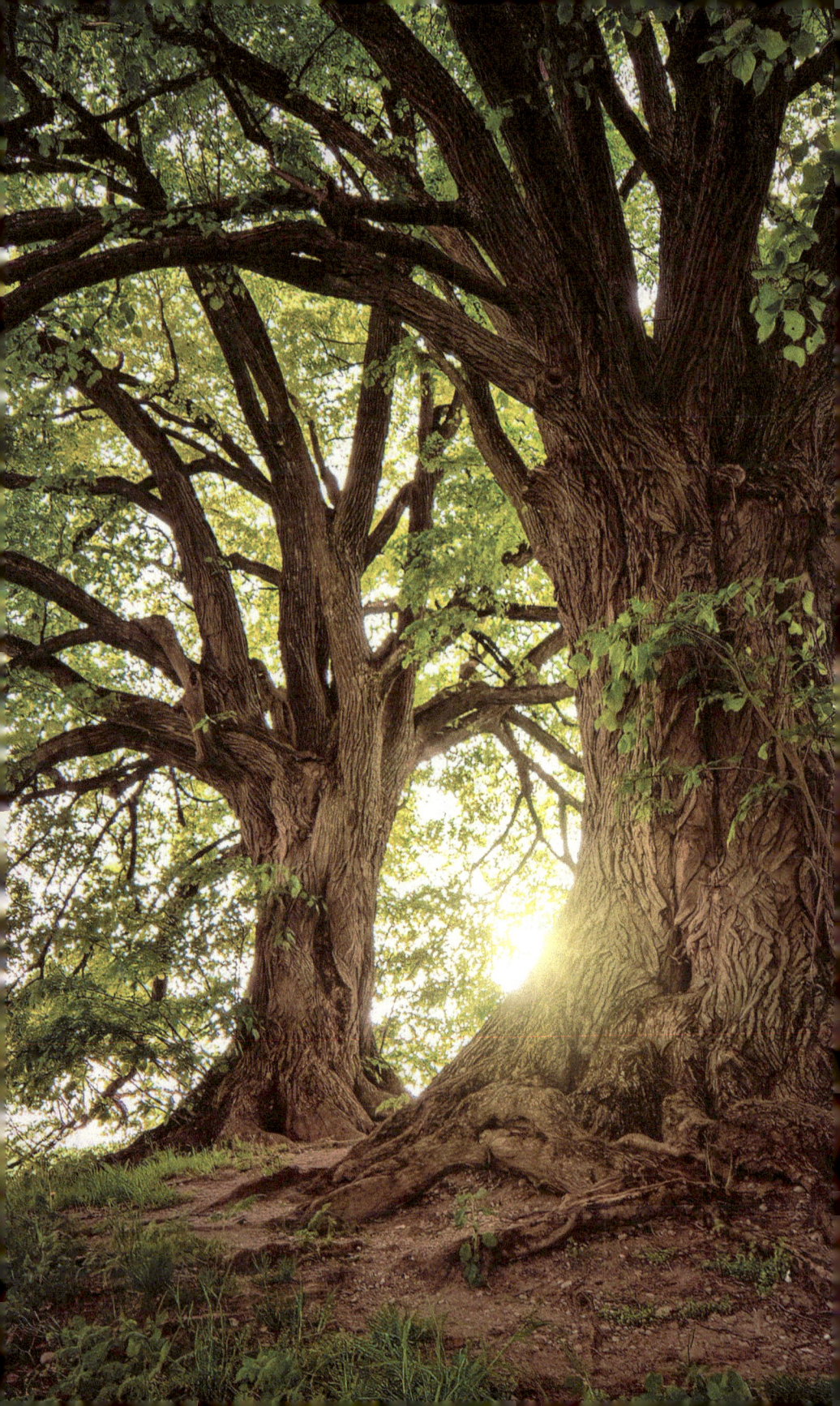

33

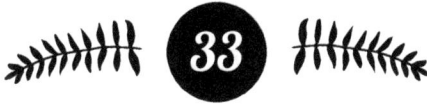

The symbol of the tree of life represents qualities like wisdom, strength, protection, beauty, bounty, and redemption. As humans, our roots are grounded by our wisdom and beliefs which grow deep. They keep us stable. Our strength and beauty branch out to bear the fruit of love, grace, and mercy. Our branches make us strong no matter what storms we weather; they are our protection. In today's prompt, take a moment and reflect on how amazingly in sync you are with your wisdom, strength, beauty, etc. and meditate on your inner tree of life. Tune into your own self-awareness. What comes up for you?

....

....

....

....

....

....

....

....

....

....

....

....

....

Oprah believes people want two things: to be seen and to be heard. I add to that and say people want to be valued and appreciated. We all want to believe we are important to someone or something. Living for a greater cause. Who or what affirmations do you seek? Is it your family? Your fans? Teachers? Your kids? Spouse? A charity? Your pets? Who or what?

....

....

....

....

....

....

....

....

....

....

....

....

....

....

....

35

Societal timelines don't mean anything! You are unlike any other person. Where you are currently is exactly where the universe designed you to be. Your testimony may help someone else. What timelines have you allowed to constrain your thoughts? Are you exactly where you thought you'd be at this time in life? If so, celebrate your wins in this next prompt. If not, write down what's missing, and why did you feel it needed to happen right now? Then cross it out and realize, you are unique.

....

....

....

....

....

....

....

....

....

....

....

....

....

....

36

Love, light, and energy. Imagine riding down the open road, windows down, sun shining, and wind fresh on your face. For me, this is when I feel most alive. Listening to my "Speak the Name" playlist I created on Spotify with great hits "You're Bigger" by Jekalyn Carr, "Speak the Name," by Koryn Hawthorne, and my favorite "The Call" by Isabel Davis—I feel joy. I feel peace. No worries, no fears, and no doubts hold me down. They all just melt away. This is where I feel the most alive. Where do you find your energy? Where do you find your peace? In what moments do you feel the most alive?

....

....

....

....

....

....

....

....

....

....

....

....

....

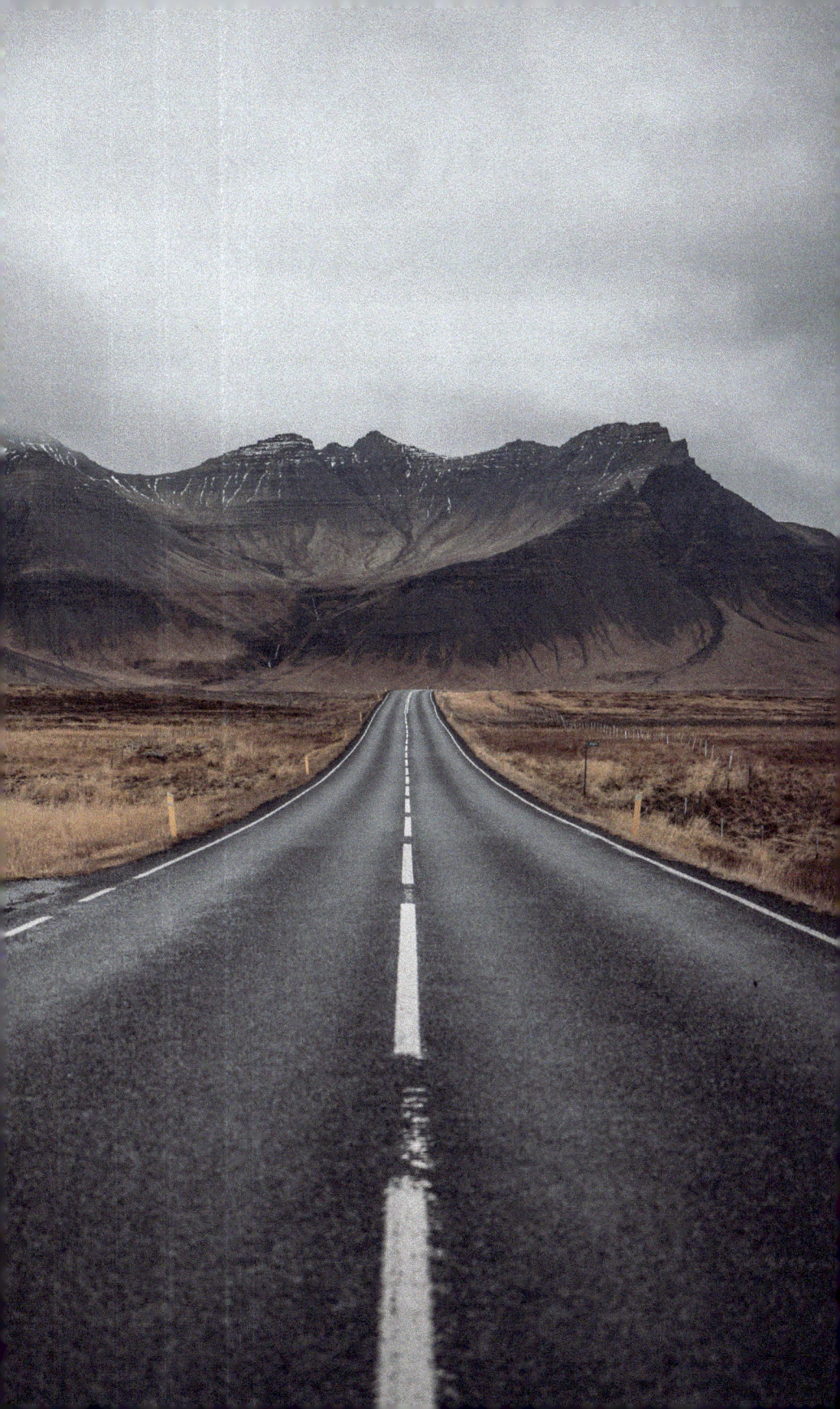

37

"Que sera, sera" means "whatever will be, will be." A song written in 1956 by Jay Livingston and Ray Evans and introduced by Doris Day still rings true today. This simple saying allows you to open your mind with curiosity and kindness. Breathe and connect in a five-minute meditation. Relax and open up by saying Que sera, sera. Whatever is happening right now in your life. Welcome the emotions. Welcome the feelings. Experience the present moment—right now, today. What is one thing you are focused on? What would it take for today to be a successful day?

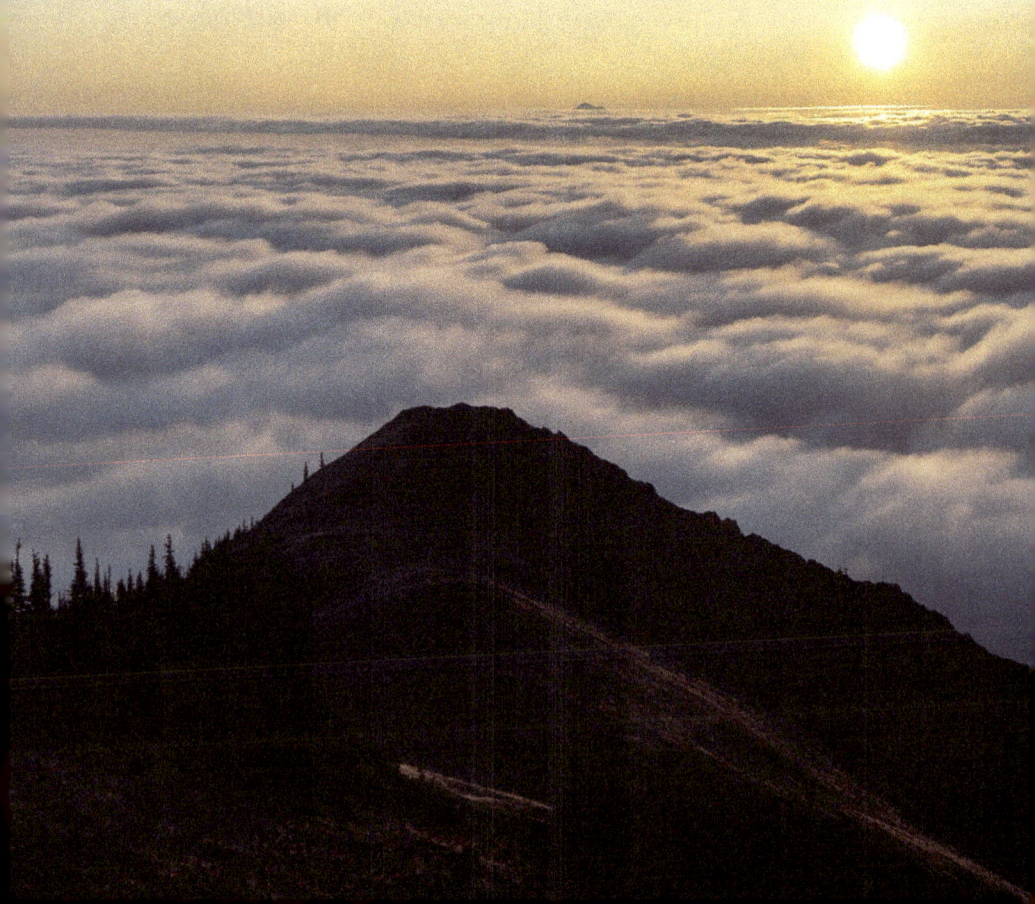

Sensation

In this next section, we'll explore emotions and senses. The idea of being present is understanding how your body reacts in certain situations. These prompts will have you step outside your comfort zone and be uncomfortable. Linger in the discomfort and explore the different emotions from the various prompts.

38

Meditative techniques for regulating body temperature are part of ancient spiritual practices. It's part of the flight or fight phenomenon in the human body. When we sense danger or fear, our body temperature often increases. Sometimes when we're angry or frustrated, sensations and pulses can be felt running through our veins. The opposite happens when we are sad or depressed. Some of us feel numb or cold. It truly is mind over matter. Think about a time when you've been upset, even if it stirs up some emotions. Now take long, deep breaths. Calm your heart rate. Switch your focus to a calming moment. Meditate on this. Did your temperature start to drop? Can you feel yourself becoming more centered? Are you now more grounded? Take a moment to write about your experience from this exercise.

....

....

....

....

....

....

....

....

....

....

....

39

I'd like for us to dive deeper into our emotions. As humans, we tend to have triggers. For me, my therapist has helped me identify my triggers and slowly work through them so they don't show up in other parts of my life. For example, when a close friend doesn't text me back in a timely manner, or if I'm not invited to a party, I normally associate this with insecurities within myself, and immediately go back to high school feelings of low self-esteem and not being good enough. You see I was bullied in High School and often ate lunch in the cafeteria bathroom because I felt so alone. It's painful to think about sometimes and I find myself in spaces where I'm always wondering whether or not I belong, or if I'm good enough for different parts of my life. Triggers can be scary sometimes, but it's when you face those fears you're able to come out stronger and grow through them. What are some triggers for you? Where do they stem from?

....

....

....

....

....

....

....

....

....

....

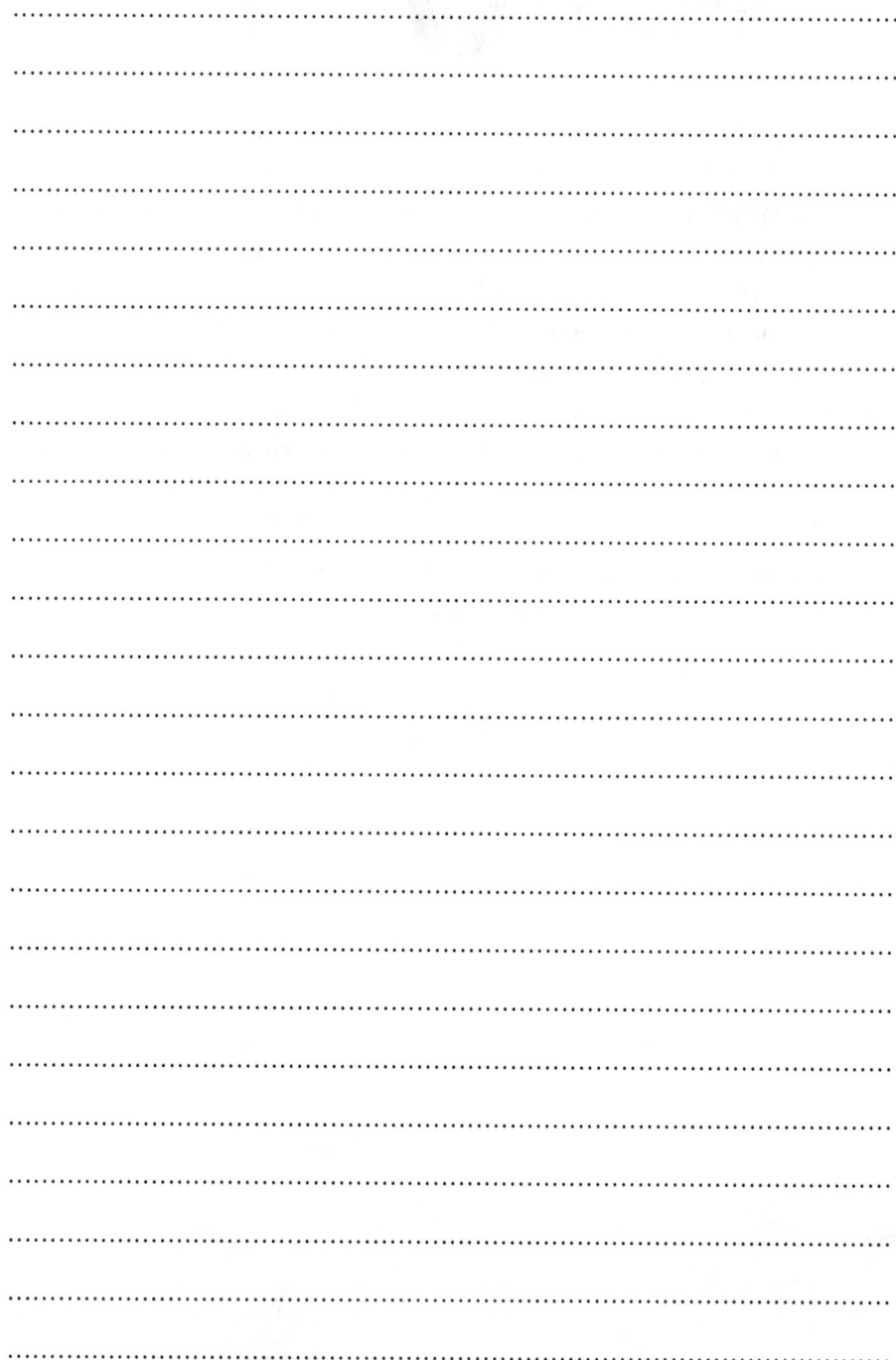

40

Emotions play an essential part in our lives. Remember a time when you were upset. What was your body's reaction? What sensations did you feel? Release the tension through paper and pen.

....

....

....

....

....

....

....

....

....

....

....

....

....

....

....

....

....

....

41

"The authentic self is soul made visible." (Sarah Ban Breathnach). Sarah, an author and public speaker, was telling us to be our authentic selves. It took me a long time to realize I'm perfectly imperfect, and I'm okay with that. I have big gums, I get loud when I'm excited, I have a sassy mouth and smile a whole lot. But I'm honest with myself and with those who come around. I don't always enjoy being vulnerable, but when I am, this allows people to see me. Recently, I've started being more vulnerable at work about racism I've experienced as a black woman all my life. From "you're not smart enough to have a Master's Degree" to "you're pretty for a dark-skinned girl." What are some negative things people or family have tried to get you to believe, and you're ready to be done with them today? What scars are still burdening your soul and you're ready to wash away?

....

....

....

....

....

....

....

....

....

....

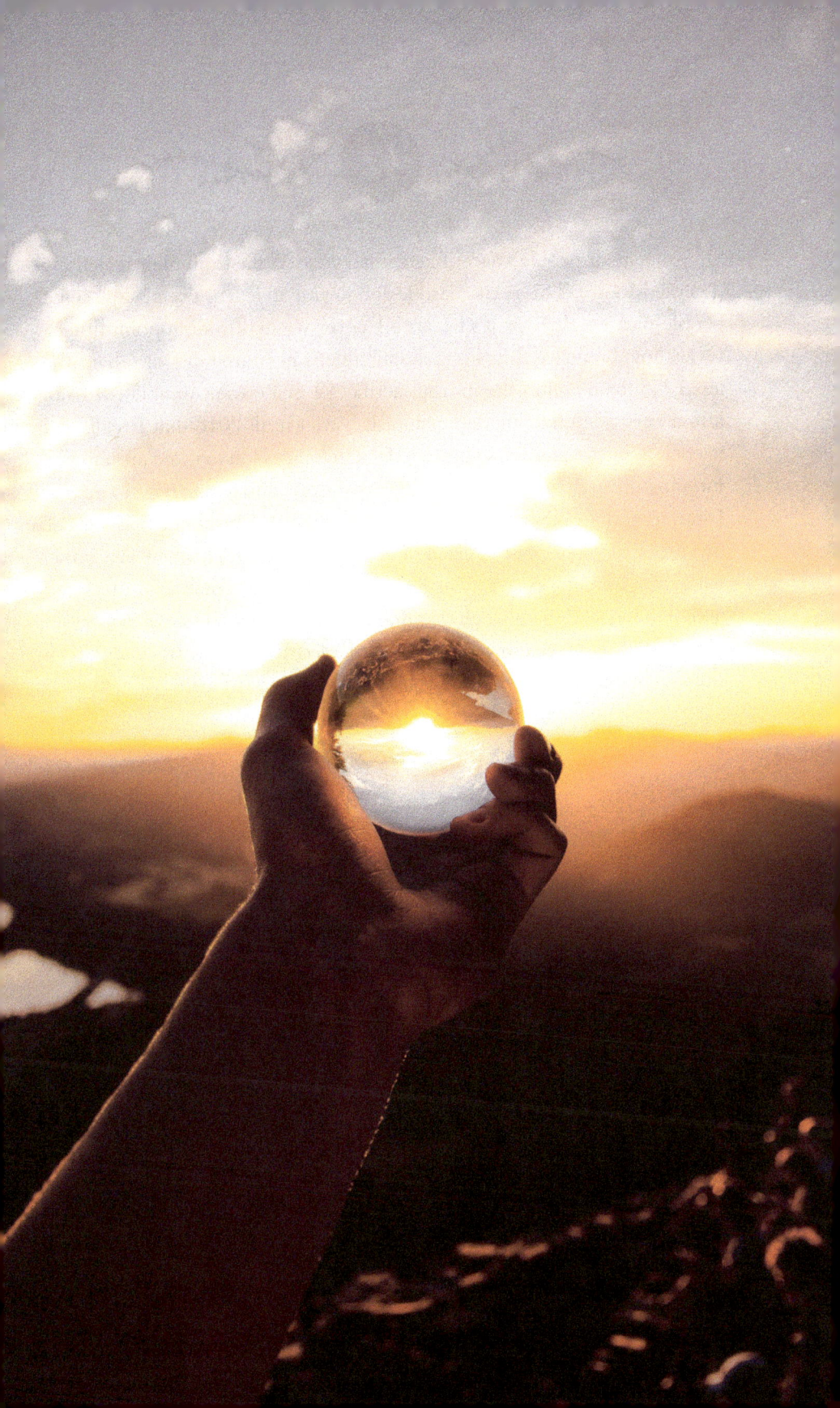

42

"If you live for people's acceptance, then you will die from their rejection" (Lecrae Moore). This was a hard lesson for me to learn. I've alway been a people-pleaser. Perhaps it's because I never wanted to disappoint others. Over time, I realized this was unsustainable. The more I did for others, the less I did for myself. Oftentimes, sacrifices I made went unnoticed. I ran into a very deep hole of depression. It wasn't until 2018 that I realized I needed to be a better me in order to be a better person to those around me. Jumping through hoops to impress everyone only did a disservice to myself. I started going to therapy, and it changed my life. I became self-aware of my gifts and talents and realized, there are people who love me for simply who I am. I was no longer vying for other people's acceptance of me. I had accepted me, and that was all that mattered. *Do you look for validity in your gifts, talents, worth, or intellectual capacity from someone or something in this world? Try a focused breathing activity then reflect on what comes up for you.*

....

....

....

....

....

....

....

....

....

43

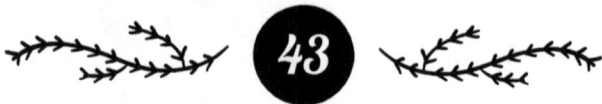

Apologizing doesn't always mean you're wrong or that the other person is right. It means you value your relationship more than your ego. In this next exercise, I want you to write an apology letter to someone you owe an apology to. Why are you apologizing? What is valuable about your relationship with that person?

....

....

....

....

....

....

....

....

....

....

....

....

....

....

....

44

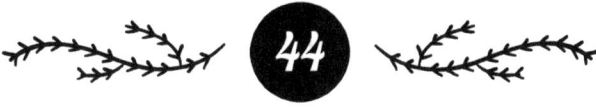

Never make any decision out of fear. What's holding you back from taking the biggest risk of your life? Sometimes our greatest risks put us in line for our biggest rewards!

....

....

....

....

....

....

....

....

....

....

....

....

....

....

....

....

....

....

45

Romans 5:3-4 says, "We can rejoice, too, when we run into problems and trials, for we know that they help us develop endurance. And endurance develops strength of character, and character strengthens our confident hope of salvation." One thing you can count on are challenges to make you stronger. I'll never forget when I had a mental breakdown at work and was overwhelmed from stress, co-workers, and customers, and I legit went into my office and cried for 20 minutes Straight. I called my dad and told him I was ready to give up. Everything was just too much for me at that moment. I'll never forget what he told me, "You will get through this, and come out stronger than you were when you started." We all have those moments where we don't think we're going to get through something and then we look back and realize wow, I made it through. That feeling of coming out on the other side is incredible. What has made you stronger? Is it a life event, a graduation, a funeral, the birth of a child? Did you overcome a hard project or season at work? Let's write about it.

....

....

....

....

....

....

....

....

....

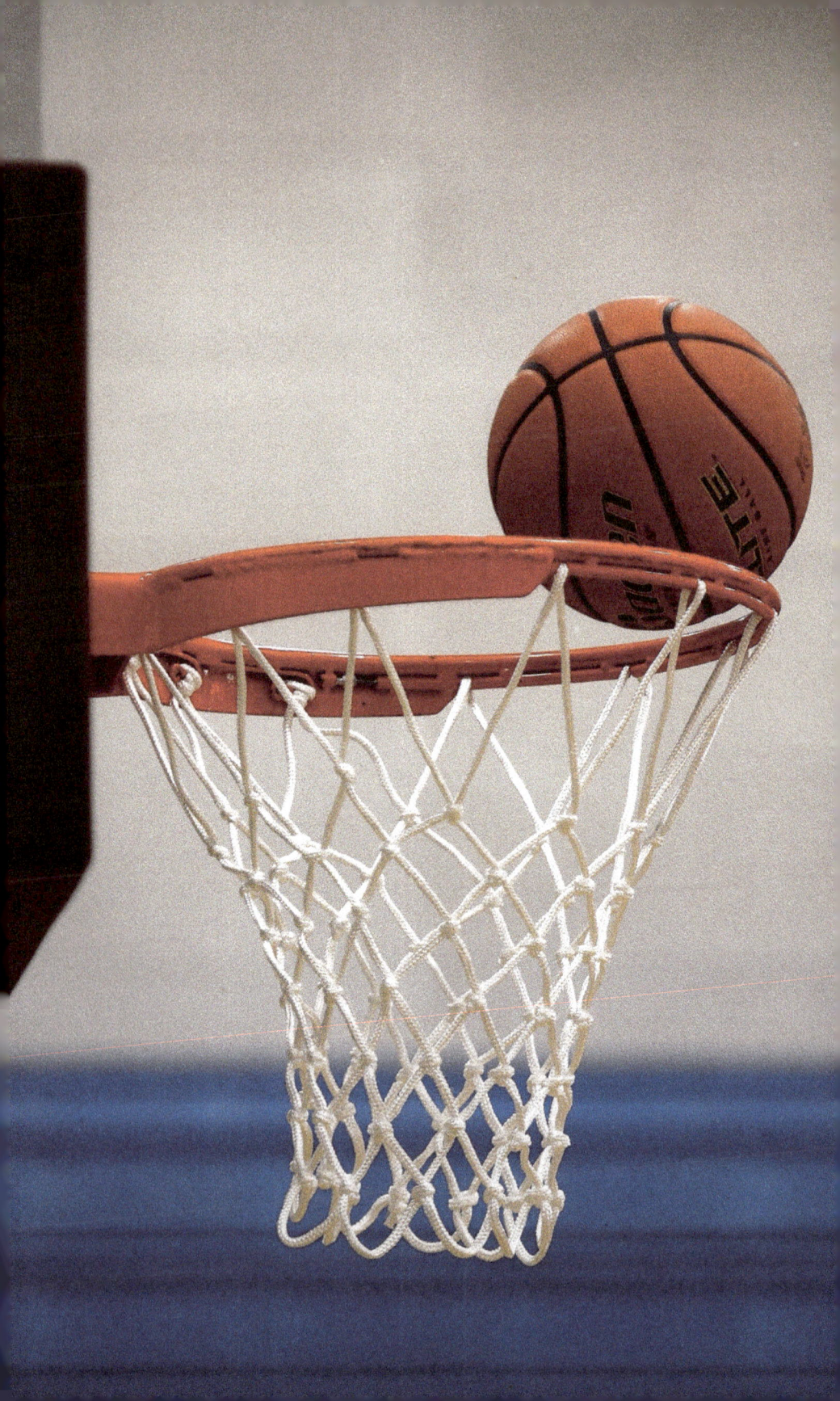

46

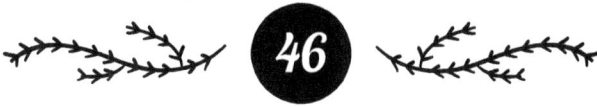

"We all have self-doubt. You don't deny it, but you also don't capitulate to it. You embrace it" (Kobe Bryant) Self-doubt is real. I can admit that, at times, I've let it overtake me more than I should have. What I've learned is that you have to get out of your head and just go for it! We miss 100 percent of the shots we don't take. Write out your self-doubts and then conquer those fears and leave them here on this page.

....

....

....

....

....

....

....

....

....

....

....

....

....

....

....

47

"If you're always trying to be normal, you will never know how amazing you can be" (Maya Angelou). Always show up and be the best version of yourself that you can be. What does the best version of yourself look like? *Try a 10-minute body scan here. Imagine your posture at each of your body parts during your scan, then come back and reflect.*

....

....

....

....

....

....

....

....

....

....

....

....

....

....

....

....

48

"Darkness cannot drive out darkness; only light can do that. Hate cannot drive out hate; only love can do that" (Martin Luther King, Jr.). I'm constantly reminded of this quote by MLK. If there's one thing I can't understand in this world, it is racism. How can you have such a disdain for someone who looks differently than you? As a black woman, I've had to deal with racism too many times in life. I'd be lying if I said this didn't affect my overall well-being and mental health. Trauma I experienced as a child is now embedded in the relationships of trust I have with people. I've learned to express my thoughts through journaling and not to allow hateful people to control my emotions. Only love can drive out such darkness. If I could change one thing about this world, it'd be to eliminate racism. If there was one thing in this world you'd change, what would it be?

....
....
....
....
....
....
....
....
....
....
....

49

"Forgiveness is giving up the hope that you could've changed the past" (Oprah Winfrey). Oftentimes, it's not easy to forgive because of the disappointment the person left with you. It took me years to forgive a close family member of mine, but I realized the longer I held on to the resentment, the more it only hurt me. I've grown to realize that in order to truly spread love and light, you need to purify your own heart and mind and welcome these emotions. A heart filled with unforgiveness for someone is a hard door to open. Be kind to yourself. Be kind to others, and forgive. Who is it you need to forgive? Reflect on who and why in this next prompt. #loveandlight

....

....

....

....

....

....

....

....

....

....

....

....

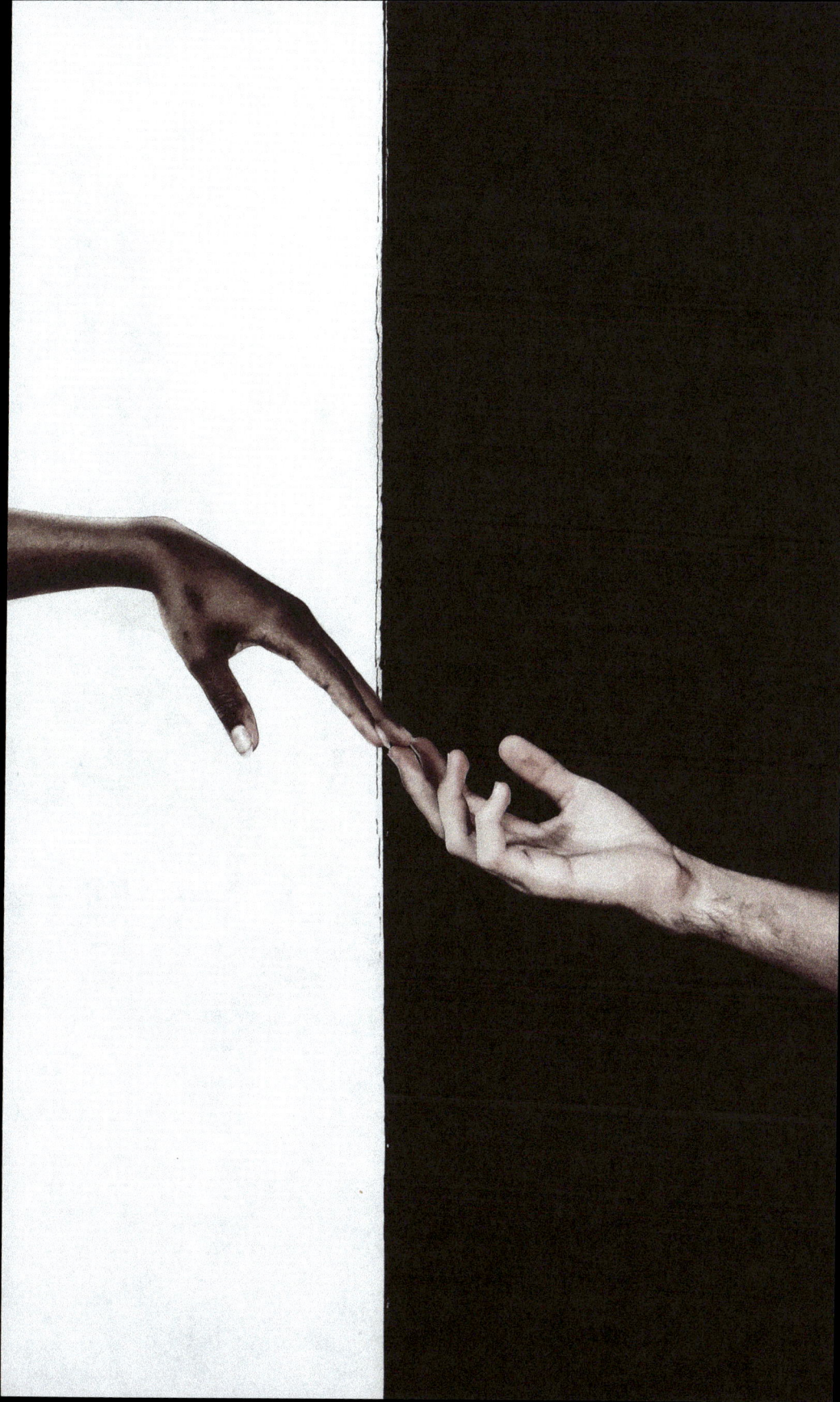

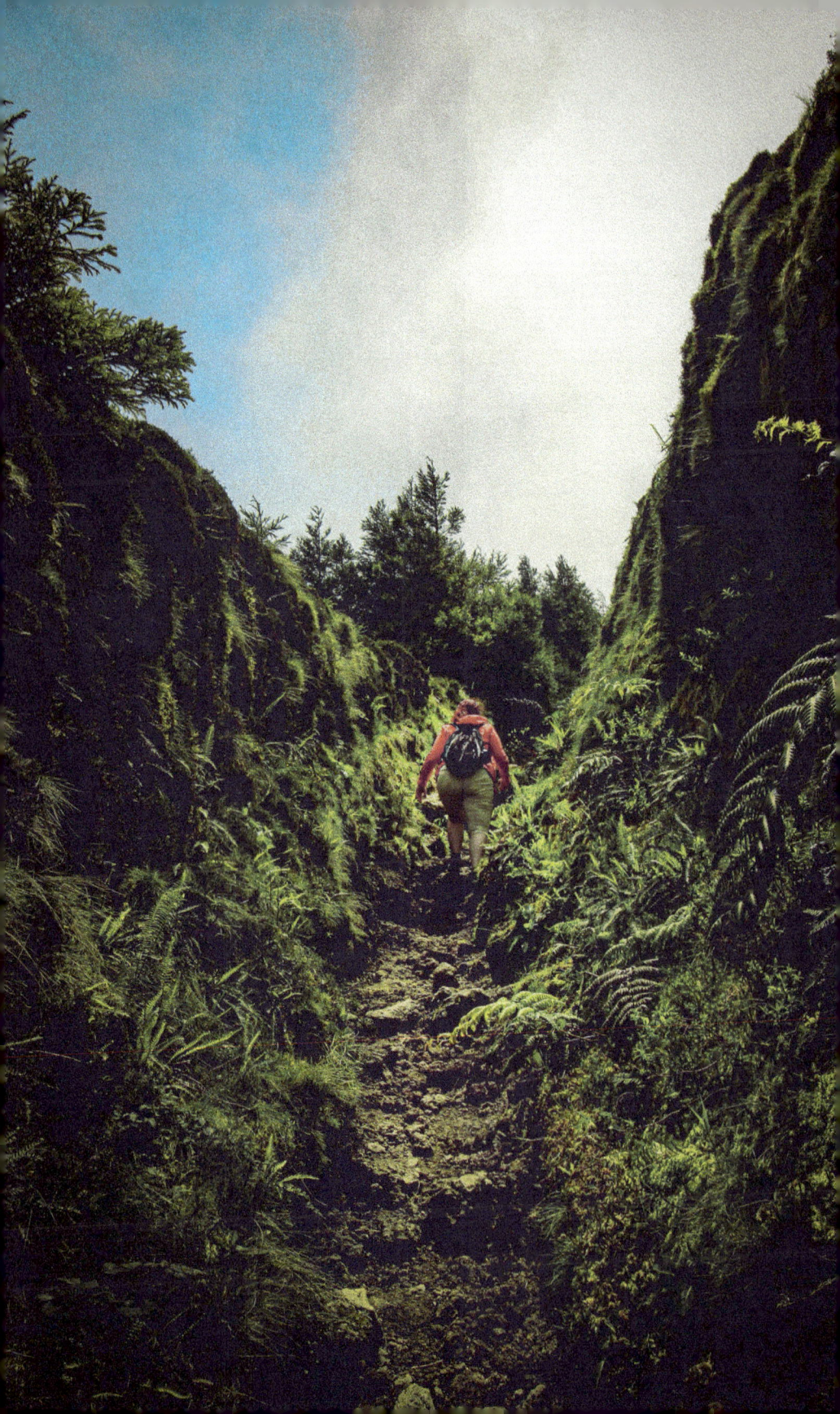

50

Don't allow others to tell you who your brand is. When someone tries to exploit your brand and image you have for yourself, look away and lean on those who support and love you. No one is perfect, and if anyone says they are... Run. This world wasn't designed for perfect people, nor for perfection. We live in a broken world with broken people who try to find the good in everyday life. In today's journal, I want you to write about a time when someone said you weren't good enough or their behaviors implied you didn't meet their expectations. What comes up for you in this reflection? Was it a job? Was it your family? Was it your children? Was it your spouse, or a friend? Who tried to tear you down, and how did you overcome it?

....

....

....

....

....

....

....

....

....

....

....

51

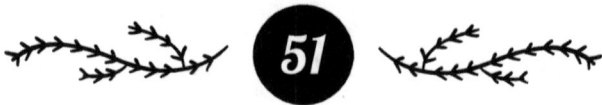

Validation is so important for us as spiritual beings. We like to be seen and to know we add value in our relationships. Make a list of people you appreciate who all want a well-balanced life of value with you.

....

....

....

....

....

....

....

....

....

....

....

....

....

....

....

....

....

....

52

Think about a time you had to overcome a challenge or a hurdle. How did you feel overcoming it? What sensations did you feel?

....

....

....

....

....

....

....

....

....

....

....

....

....

....

....

....

....

....

....

53

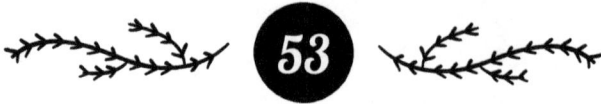

Time is the one currency you can't get back. Own it! You are valuable. Stop wasting your time and energy on things or people who don't add value to your life. Take one minute to meditate and focus on where you'd like to remove your time and energy. Which relationships, events, or things don't deserve your time and energy? Then come back and refocus on where you would like to expend your energy.

....

....

....

....

....

....

....

....

....

....

....

....

....

....

54

"My life is mines" (Tracey Ellis Ross). Where are places you feel you aren't living your life? What are some areas you feel like you're wearing a mask or barely holding your head above water sometimes? When I first heard Tracey speak those four little words, how simple. *"My life,"* all of the trauma I've been through, hurt I've experienced has made me who I am today. It's allowed me to fail fast and corset correct when necessary. *"Is mines,"* no matter what flaws I see in myself, I own them and they make me stronger. I've experienced racism, discrimination, a broken heart, low self-esteem, being bullied, and each time, I've come out swimming. It's on the other side of those moments, you realize you're an absolute badass! Don't allow your past to hold you in guilt, shame or hurt. Embrace the idea that "My life is mines."

....
....
....
....
....
....
....
....
....
....
....

55

Some of our darkest places will bring out our most meaningful messages and lessons. It's from these places we discover our strength through tension. It is that, my friend, which allows us to reach our full potential. Take a moment to reflect on a moment or a season where you didn't think you'd be able to come back from. What are the lessons you learned during those times? What did you learn about yourself? For me, it was when I started my first job straight out of grad school. I was the youngest manager at my company and constantly told I didn't fit the corporate culture. I didn't have the corporate speak down just yet, my salary wasn't enough to keep me in designer clothes, and I was still driving the car my parents got me when I graduated from undergrad. Even when so many around doubted me, I surrounded myself with people who believed in me. I kept showing up. I didn't stop. Did I get down some days? Sure. But I was determined to get through my struggle. I ended up working for the company for five years, being promoted, and I outlasted three different managers. I became an expert in my field. The experience made me stronger, I proved to myself that I'm not a quitter. I'm so thankful for that time in my career because now when I have haters in my life, it's easier to recognize them and respond differently. What's your story and lesson you've overcome?

....

....

....

....

....

....

Transformation

Be the change you want to see! These next few prompts will focus on areas of growth and maturation. We'll explore prompts related to your current events and future goals. In order to achieve transformation and triumph you must first explore what makes you well.

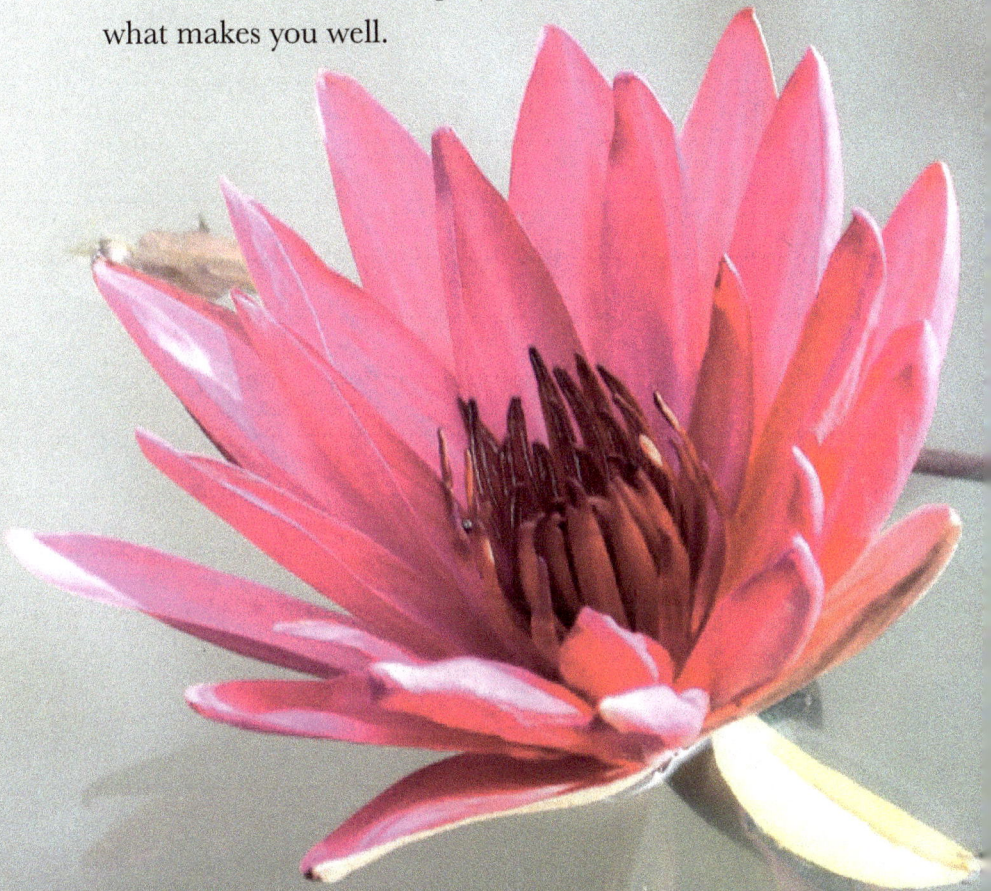

56

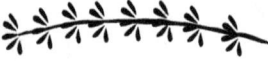

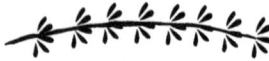

Benchmark where you are, then acknowledge your growth. In order to measure where we want to be, we must first acknowledge where we are. Consider this moment as a "You Are Here." What are some things you've been able to accomplish in the last six months? Now what areas do you want to focus on for the next six months? For example, I've been exploring a lot more in the kitchen. Finding new recipes to try out and sharing with my neighbors. I've also decided to learn SQL (a programming language). I've been inconsistent and need to practice more, but that'll be my focus over the next six months. Benchmark where you are and grow from there.

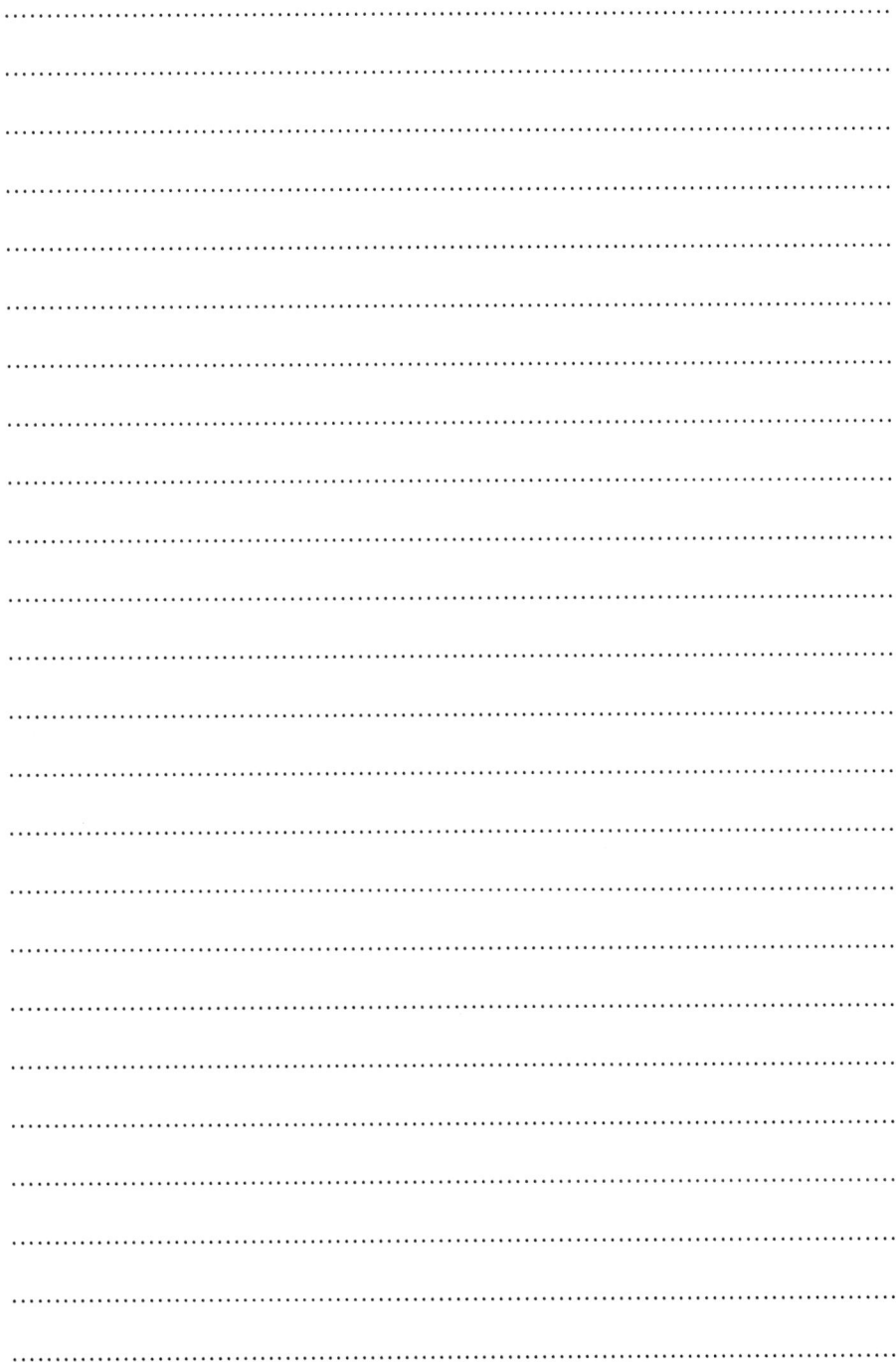

57

F.O.C.U.S. = Forget Obstacles Circumventing Underlying Situations. What is holding you back from pushing forward? Don't let anything stand in the way of your greatness. Stay focused! How are you going to stay focused this week? Here are some of my suggestions: 1. Meditation 2. Unplug from social media, the TV or your computer. 3. Hire a babysitter for an hour so you can really focus on you.

....

....

....

....

....

....

....

....

....

....

....

....

....

....

....

58

Focus: Manifest your Destiny. For one week, create a to-do list, and knock out everything on that list. Circle back to this prompt and see how productive your week ended. Don't overwhelm yourself. Start with small wins. Pretty soon, those wins will turn into large victories. These habits will help you start manifesting your destiny into a reality.

....
....
....
....
....
....
....
....
....
....
....
....
....
....
....
....

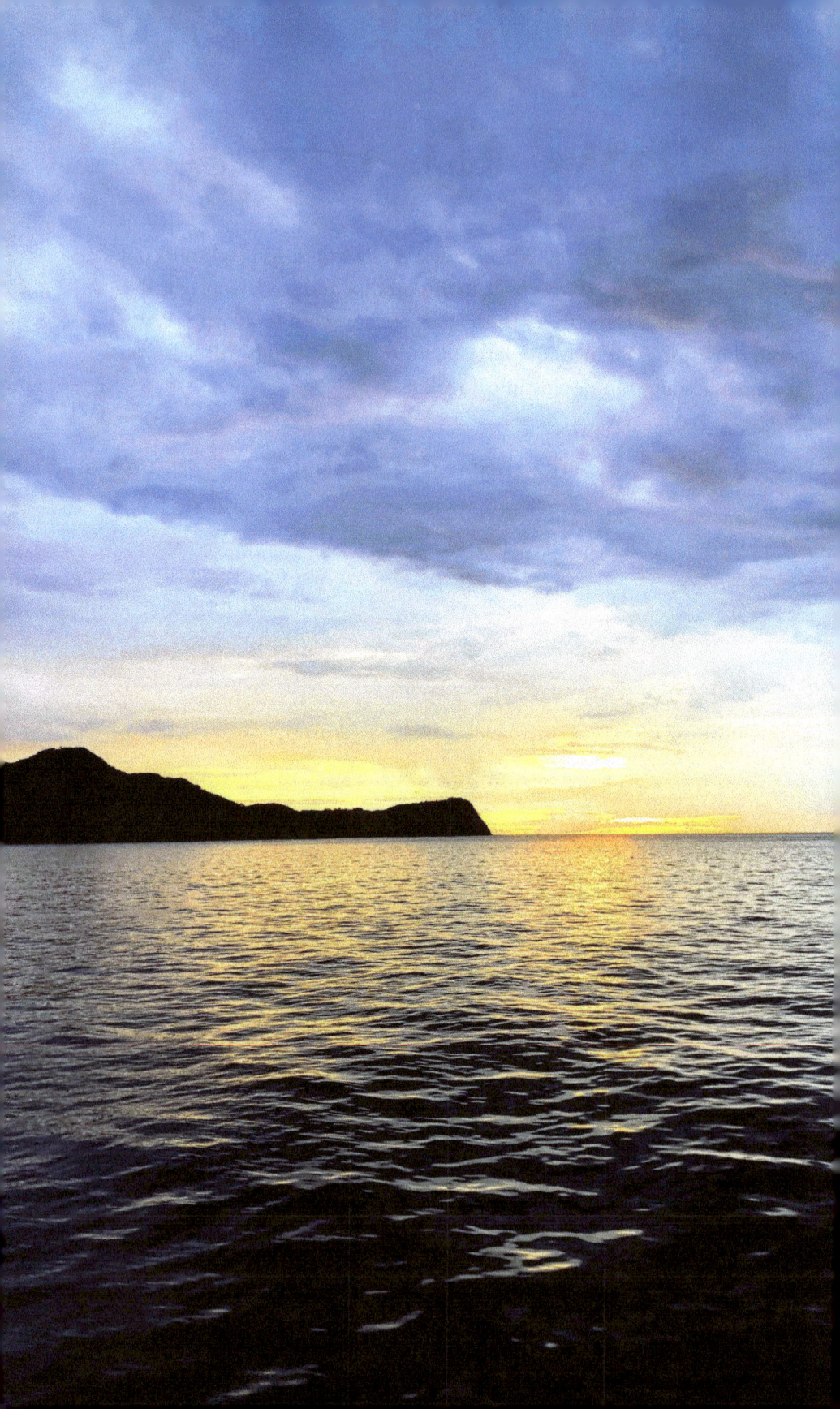

59

"An intention is the first whisper of purpose you bring to what you do or say. It's the real motivation behind any action. The why behind the why." (Oprah Winfrey). The energy which drives your motivation is what determines your outcome. What's your why? Why have you chosen to embark on a journey of wellness? What's motivating you down this path.

....
....
....
....
....
....
....
....
....
....
....
....
....
....
....
....
....

60

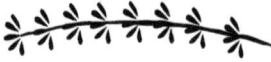

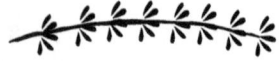

Growing up, I often heard people say "you have a childlike innocence." Many times, I was offended by such a comment because I felt people were saying I was young or immature. Now, when I hear this expression, I have a different outlook; it means I like to keep things simple and light. Children are far more curious and creative than some adults I know. It's that curiosity mindset that allows them to explore this world unbothered and so fearless. In today's prompt, imagine a younger you. Take a day and explore the world through a child's lens. Where would you go and what would you do? Do you want to go to a park and play or would you rather stay home and build a fort with pillows and sheets? The world is your oyster. Have fun with this prompt and let the pen guide you.

61

It's better to have loved than to never have loved at all. Love is one of the most powerful forces in this world. People have eloped for love. People have ravaged territories for love. People go on reality TV for love. It's an action that drives some people to do the unthinkable. The love we have for our families and friends — the time and energy we invest — is so great. The world needs more love. My family, friends, and spouse remind me that community and compassion for others fuels me. It's the love for these people which inspires me and motivates me to wake up each and every day and do my best. How has love impacted your life today?

....

....

....

....

....

....

....

....

....

....

....

....

....

62

In 2020, people saw unprecedented times. We were reminded that tomorrow isn't always promised. The social isolation, closing of stores, cancellations of major sports, concerts, and festivals have all shown us that we're not always promised tomorrow, so live for the moment. As part of a society which is always on the go, COVID-19 allowed me personally to take a step back and remember what truly matters. No matter what season you're in — from losing a job to moving somewhere new — what is the most important part of life for you? Which values follow you through every season? *Pause and reflect. What values lie close to your heart?*

....

....

....

....

....

....

....

....

....

....

....

....

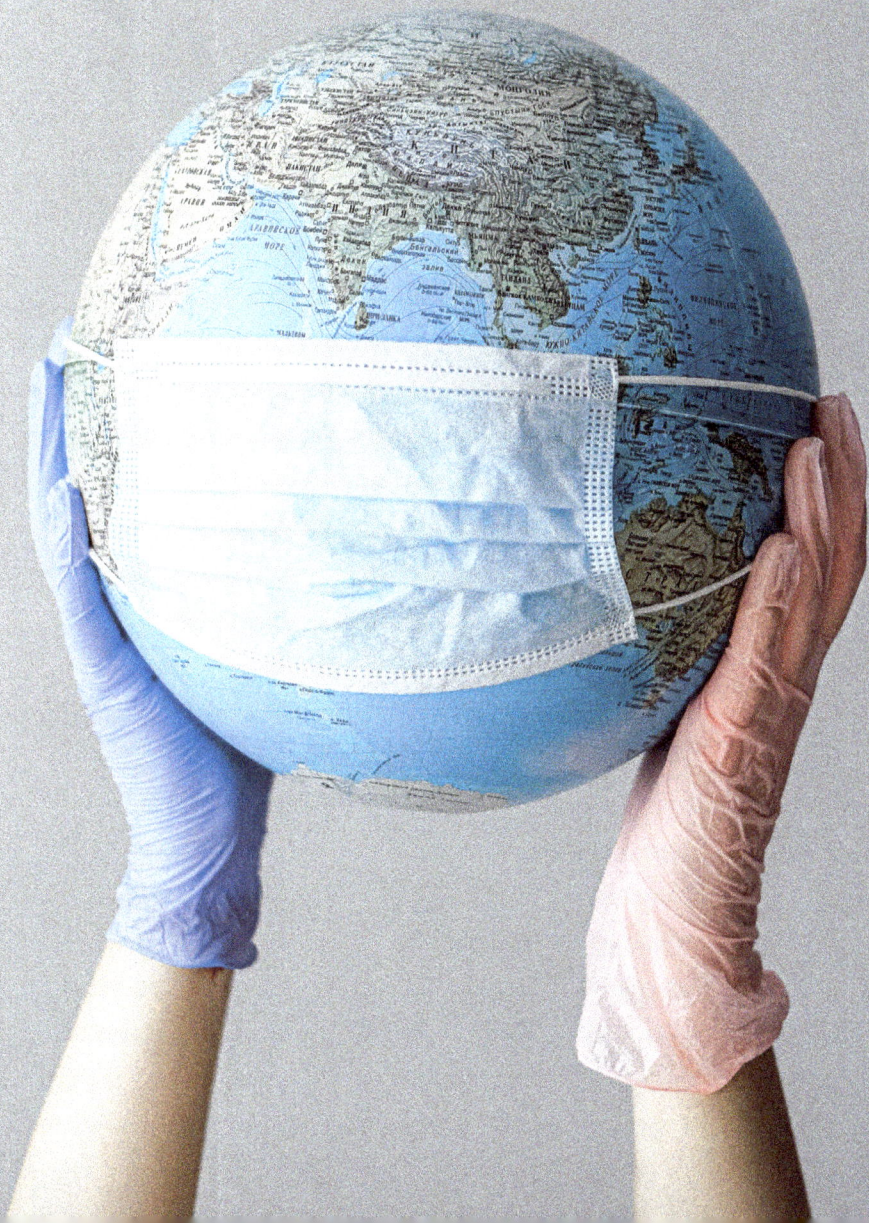

63

It's not about the number of years you live on this earth, but how you fill those years. What do you want to be remembered for and by whom? Define your legacy.

....

....

....

....

....

....

....

....

....

....

....

....

....

....

....

....

....

64

It doesn't cost anything to be kind. Close your eyes. Listen to your breathing for two minutes. Imagine the last time you were kind. What did you feel at that moment? Who benefited from your kindness?

....

....

....

....

....

....

....

....

....

....

....

....

....

....

....

....

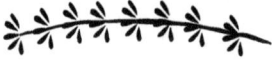

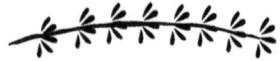

Continuing our notion of kindness. Remember, it pays to be kind. Often-times I've found when I was down, or feeling unmotivated, the act of doing something to put a smile on someone else's face has made me feel better. For example, I've sent flowers to my best friend, paid a compliment to my co-worker in the office. Sometimes I cook my spouse his favorite dinner and it brings joy to my heart. What's one small act you can do today to show kindness?

....

....

....

....

....

....

....

....

....

....

....

....

....

66

I took a training class and my instructor had us write down where we wanted to be in one year. At first it was odd to think about because we needed to describe our day in so much detail. However, it was the first time I felt so free to be me. I wrote how I'd like to be on the beach, waking up to the waves, a chef making me breakfast and making business calls while overlooking an ocean. It was incredible. It was also motivation to work toward that ideal day for my future. Imagine yourself waking up a year from today. Where are you? Who are you with? Write in the present tense as you live out that day. If you aren't there in a year, start today in making a plan to get there one day. Use this as your motivation. Think of it as your North star.

....

....

....

....

....

....

....

....

....

....

....

....

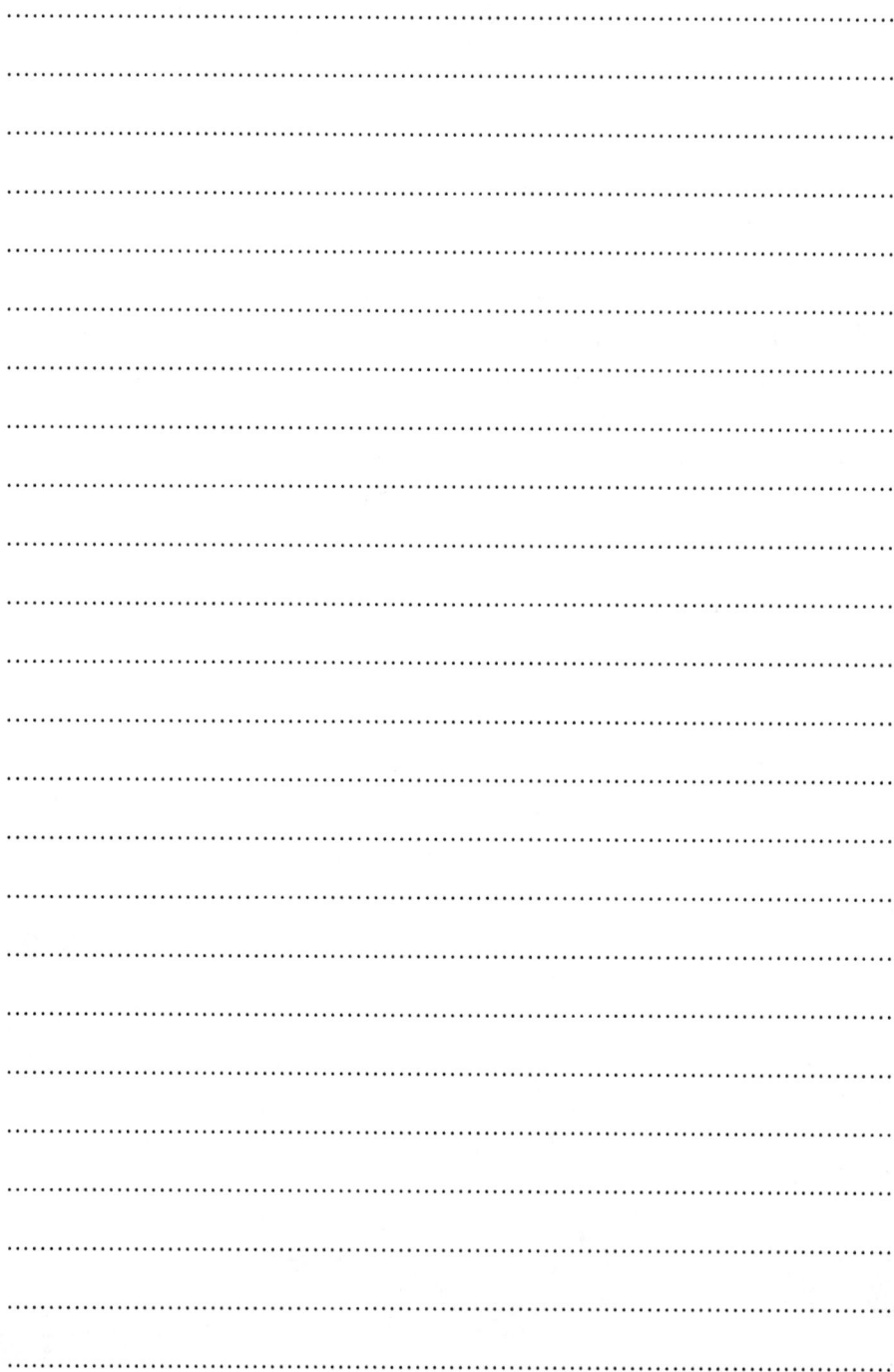

67

Patience is a virtue. Life is a gift. Take a moment to reflect on those you consistently want to give your presence to.

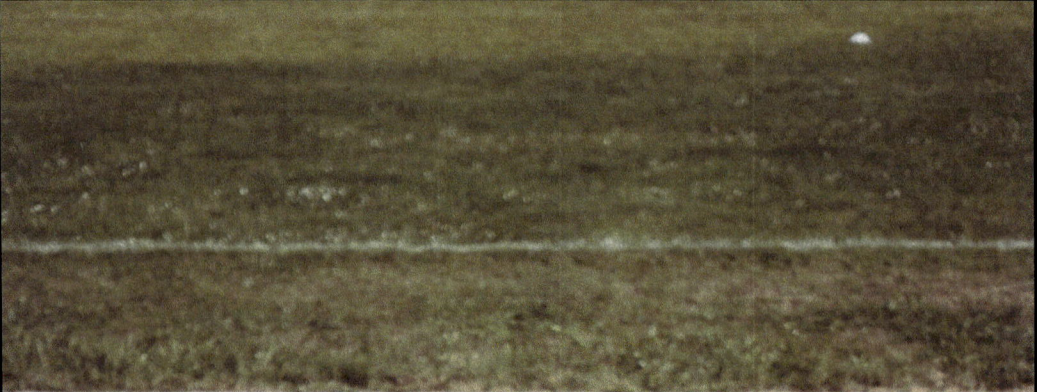

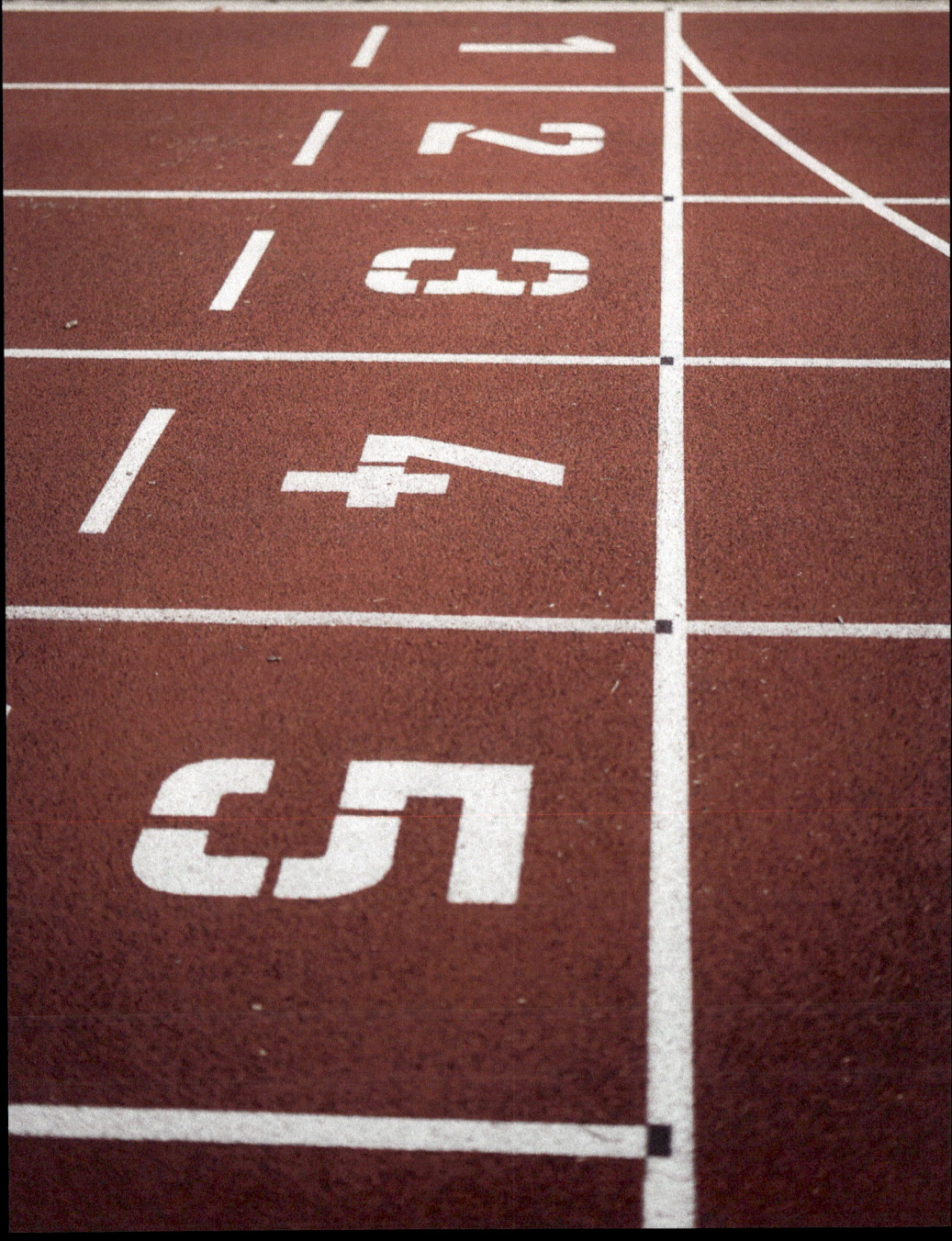

68

I want to remind you that getting through this book is a marathon, not a sprint. Being intentional in our lives is very important. So be intentional about your thoughts, feelings, and answers to the prompts. It is only through our intentions that we start to change our actions, behaviors, and life overall. What were your initial intentions when starting this journey? Have those intentions changed? Have they evolved? Reflect on what's remained the same and what's changed.

....
....
....
....
....
....
....
....
....
....
....
....
....
....

69

Keep doing you! Let's write about it. How would you define who you are? When people look at you, what do they see? What do you want them to see? The most important thing to know is YOU are an amazing, awesome person. So BE you! And keep doing you!

....
....
....
....
....
....
....
....
....
....
....
....
....
....
....
....

70

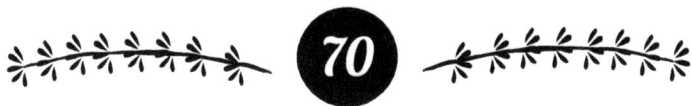

"Never be limited by other people's imaginations" (Dr. Mae Jemison). Your life's purpose and meaning is ultimately decided by your attitude and the output you choose to put into the universe. Take a minute to write down your most far-fetched idea or dream.

....
....
....
....
....
....
....
....
....
....
....
....
....
....
....
....
....

71

F.E.A.R.= Forget Everyone Around you and Run towards your destiny! We can't be afraid of our fears. We must conquer our fears and persevere! What's a fear you want to conquer this year?

....

....

....

....

....

....

....

....

....

....

....

....

....

....

....

....

....

72

"Comparison is the thief of joy" (Theodore Roosevelt). Social media and the increase in mental health issues shouldn't come as a shock as this generation is often faced with comparisons. Remain true to yourself. Take a moment and reflect what or who you constantly compare yourself to. Use this time to let it out.

....

....

....

....

....

....

....

....

....

....

....

....

....

....

....

....

....

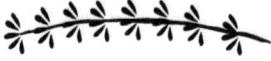

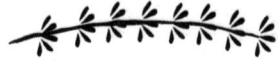

Our attitude determines our altitude. Your thoughts determine how you approach life. Picture your mind as a mountain. The more positive thoughts you create within yourself, the higher you're able to climb on the mountain. We should always be striving to be a better version of the person we were yesterday. Draw a mountain and write down things you want to reach at each level. For example, I want to get better at playing guitar. I want to learn another language. I want to be a better friend. I want to learn a new skill. Determine how tall you want your mountain to be and remember your attitude will determine how high you climb that mountain.

....

....

....

....

....

....

....

....

....

....

....

....

....

74

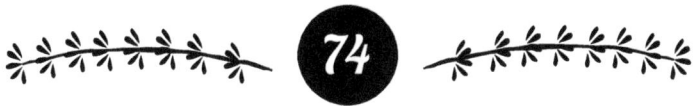

Positive energy put out into the universe brings back good Karma. Are you focused on a positive attitude? Share an area where this is paying off.

....

....

....

....

....

....

....

....

....

....

....

....

....

....

....

....

....

....

75

"Our deepest fear is not that we are inadequate. Our deepest fear is that we are powerful beyond measure. It is our light, not our darkness that most frightens us" (Marianne Williamson). I heard this quote while at the Oprah Vision 2020 tour. I wanted to include this in my book because I do truly believe we are powerful beyond measure. On my wellness journey, I've started to embrace the here and now. If there's greatness happening in my life, I want to explore it. I want to celebrate it with those I love and people who are supportive of my happiness. When there's tension in my life, I used to want to hide away in a dark room. I'd become lonely and depressed. Now, I ask myself what am I supposed to learn at this moment? Why have the stars aligned with these complications for me to face? What is the lesson I'm meant to learn here? How can I share this story with someone later? I encourage you to latch on to this same belief. Ask yourself: what is life giving you right now and what is the lesson to celebrate? Good, bad, and everything in between.

76

"Intention makes you pay attention" (Ricki Wax). It's happening whether you realize it or not. Every action has a reaction. So you get what you put into life to get what you want out of life. What are you putting out today?

77

Repeat after me: My daily decisions must be met with constant choices which align with my well thought-out intentions in order for me to feel successful. Each day brings forth new opportunities to change who I am becoming. I can't always change the circumstances in front of me, but I do have the power to change the way I respond. I have the power to change my mindset. I have the power to only change myself. Who are you becoming?

....
....
....
....
....
....
....
....
....
....
....
....
....
....

78

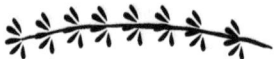

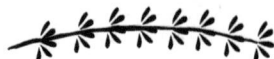

In this next prompt, I want us to revisit our acronym we learned. F.O.C.U.S.: Forget. Obstacles. Circumventing. Underlying. Situations. Focus your mind on what you want to happen. I recently started listening to deep focus concentration music. A colleague of mine recommended it while I was leading a "Mindful Moments" session. I normally have my go-to playlists, so this was definitely something new and fresh for me to try. Fast-forward three weeks, and I find the music to be very soothing while I work. I'm not distracted by song lyrics or someone's voice. It really helps me get into a zone and be productive. Check out Spotify or Youtube, and try listening to a concentration playlist while writing. *Journal one of your favorite topics which has been discussed so far in your wellness journey.*

....

....

....

....

....

....

....

....

....

....

....

....

FOCUS

Forget
Obstacles
Circumventing
Underlying
Situations

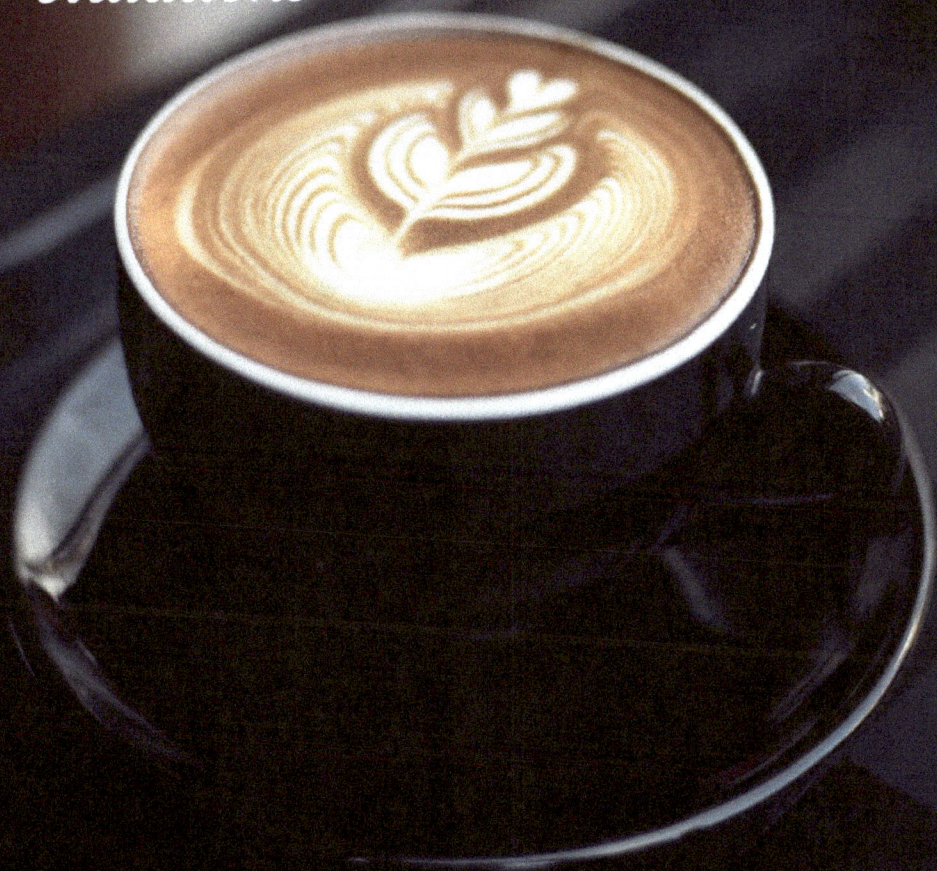

79

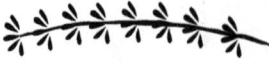

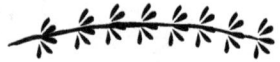

Shower Meditation. In today's exercise, I want you to meditate in the shower. For some, this is our only time alone, away from family, the kids, or our spouses. It's such a nice sanctuary in our home. I enjoy listening to the water hit the floor and splash around my feet. Seeing the steam rise from my hands to the ceiling. Feeling the hot water grace my skin. It's such an intimate moment, yet we rush through it oftentimes as a means to an end. For today's prompt, I want you to practice mindful meditation in the shower. *Observe the sounds, focus on the objects in the shower, silence your thoughts, and inhale the steam. Enjoy just being. Come back and reflect how this shower was different from most in your journal exercise once done.*

80

Start each day with a grateful heart. This next exercise should be an easy and fun thing to do. You're going to write a letter to yourself explaining things you are grateful for and congratulate yourself on your milestones. These can be big or small. I'll help you get started. *Dear journal, Today I am grateful for my health, my friends, and my family. I'm grateful to be surrounded by my biggest cheerleader, my partner and spouse. We celebrate three months in our first home!* Now you try.

....

....

....

....

....

....

....

....

....

....

....

....

....

....

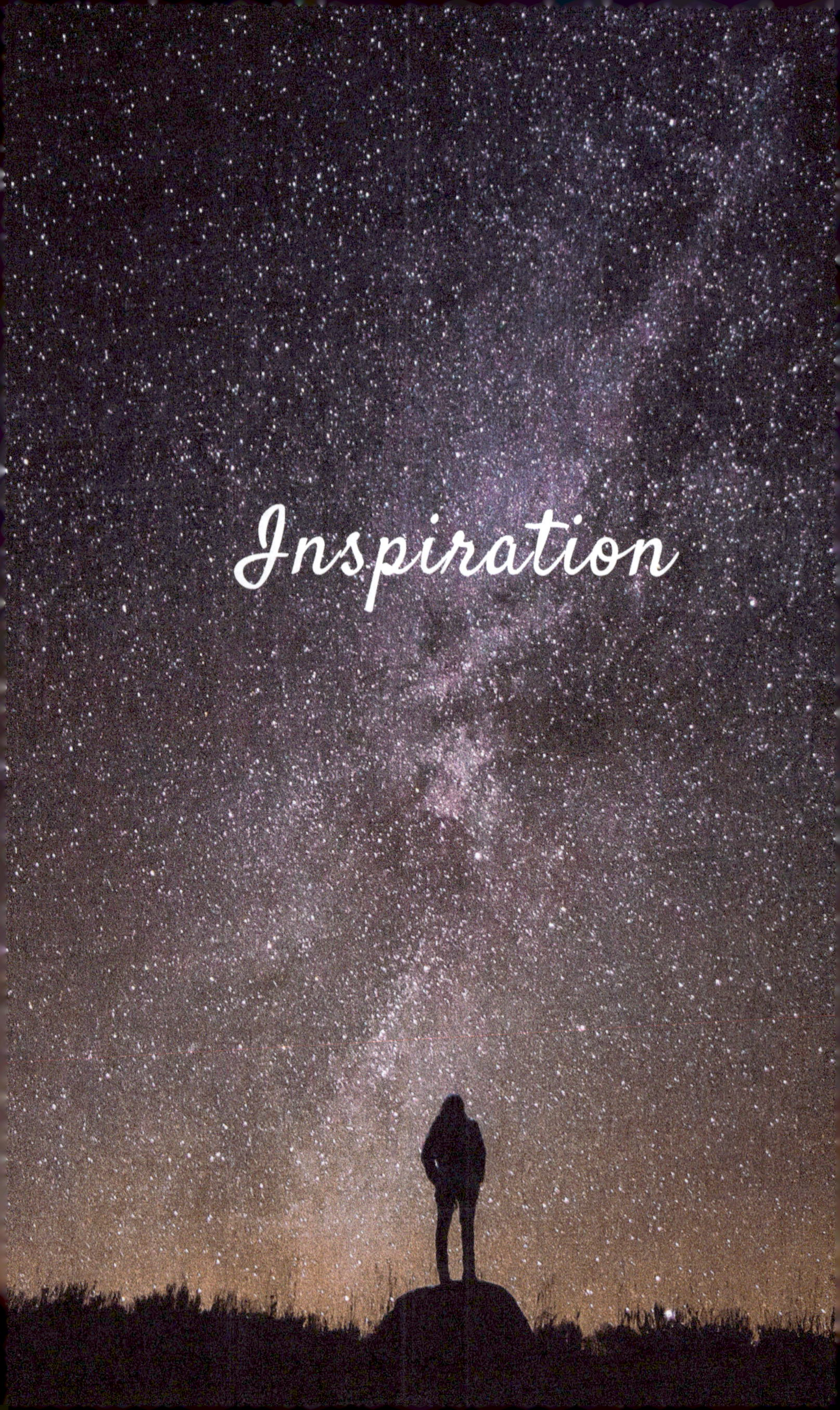

Inspiration

As we round out our last section of our journal. I wanted to end on a high note of inspirational prompts. These prompts will explore your purpose and passion. I've designed them to invoke excitement in your future. A key piece of advice as you explore this section is to ask yourself, do I need to wait for one day or can I make this day one?

81

"Use your signature strengths and virtues in the service of something much larger than you are" (Martin Seligman). Today, let's reflect on your strengths. What are some areas you excel in? Now focus on how you can use those for good.

82

What's one habit you can start today to help you on your path toward living a more mindful life?

....
....
....
....
....
....
....
....
....
....
....
....
....
....
....
....
....

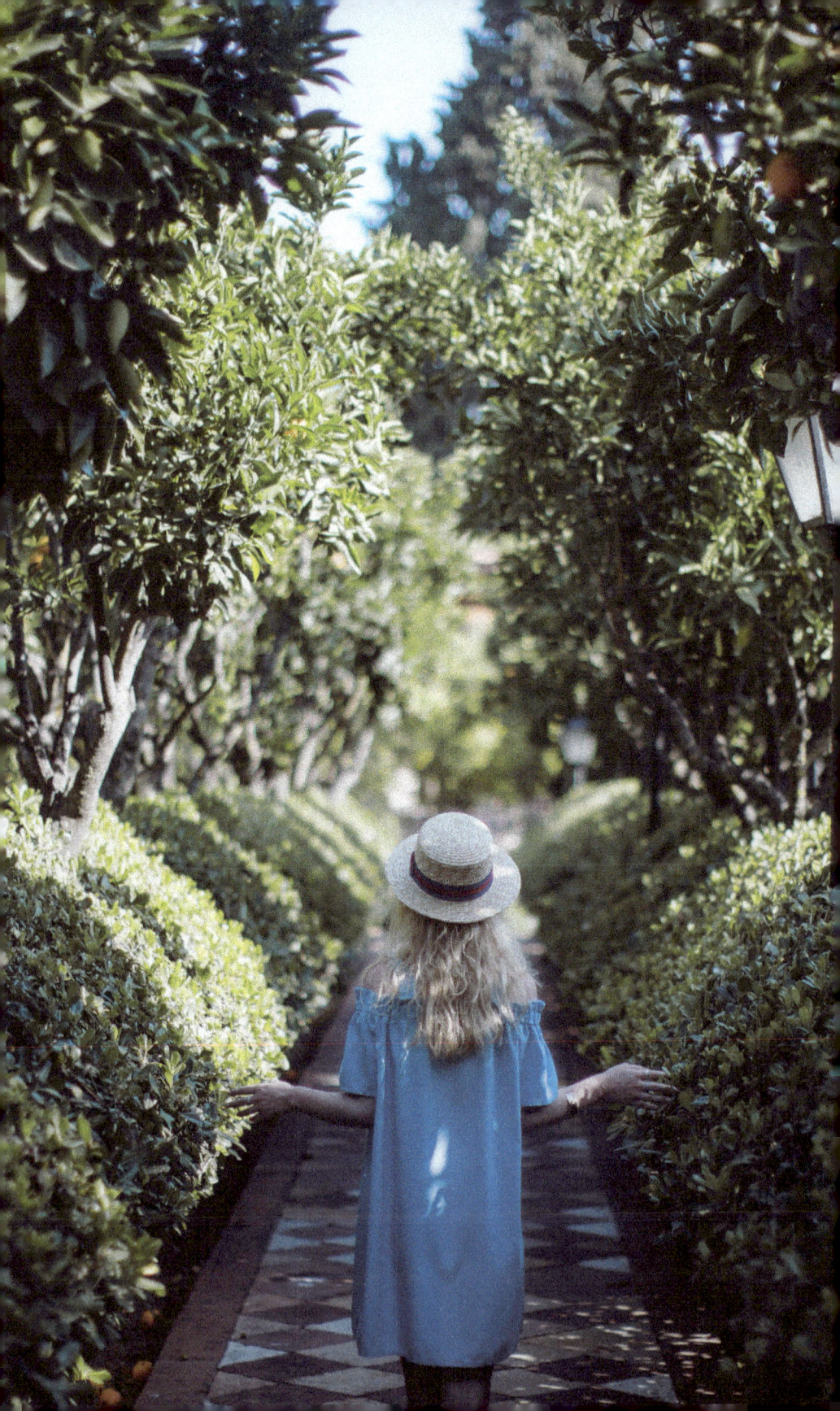

83

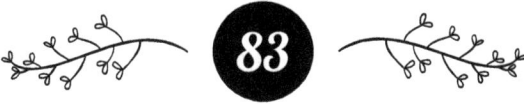

Wellness is a practice which leads to your best life. Take a mindful walk in nature and allow the outdoors to energize you. Remember mindful walking is being intentional in each step. For me, I like to hear the grass crunching under my feet, the wind sweeping across my face; I spread my arms to feel the heat on my skin and recharge me. Mindfulness leads to a life of well-being which allows you to lead your best life. Reflect on your mindful walk today. What recharged you? Describe the scenery in detail.

....

....

....

....

....

....

....

....

....

....

....

....

....

84

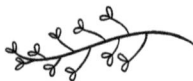

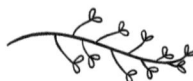

I once had someone wise tell me, "happiness is a fleeting feeling. Instead, we should strive for content and purpose." There's absolutely nothing wrong with feeling happiness, because without happiness, we do not know sadness. However, I challenge you to strive for purpose and contentment in order to achieve life satisfaction. In this next prompt, take a second to visit your happy place. Where do you go? What do you see? Describe each aspect in detail. The smell, sounds, temperature, your body posture, and state of mind at your happy place.

85

Pursue your passion. As we continue to reflect on how to optimize living a fulfilling life, let's rediscover your passion. The best advice I ever received was: "Your passion is something you can talk about without even thinking about it. It comes easy to you. It excites you. It's okay to be passionate about more than one thing." These next few sections will allow you to become more in tune with what your passion(s) are. What comes easy to you?

....

....

....

....

....

....

....

....

....

....

....

....

....

....

86

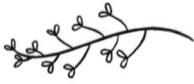

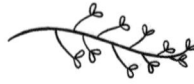

Reflect. Passion vs. Purpose. I've had many discussions with my friends on passion and purpose. If you're lucky, some of us are able to live out our purpose in our everyday jobs and in those spaces we've carved out our passion. However, some separate the two paths altogether. For me, I'm still on a journey to where I embed my passion into my work. I am an avid volunteer and board member mentee for nonprofits, which help support my passion to causes benefitting underrepresented groups. By putting my passion into my work and weaving my extracurricular activities into my life, I often feel like I'm living up to my purpose. Take a mindful walk today and ask yourself: am I living in my purpose? Have I discovered my passion? Then come back and journal what came up for you.

....

....

....

....

....

....

....

....

....

....

....

....

87

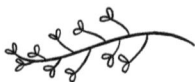

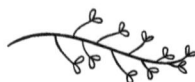

Good leaders lift as you climb. In workshops I lead, I always tell my students: once you feel you've reached a level of success defined by yourself, always pay it forward. Meaning, continue to help develop others, scope out opportunities which may have future leaders, share access to resources which can benefit those around you. This demonstrates true leadership. Name three ways you are currently paying it forward or would like to pay it forward in the future.

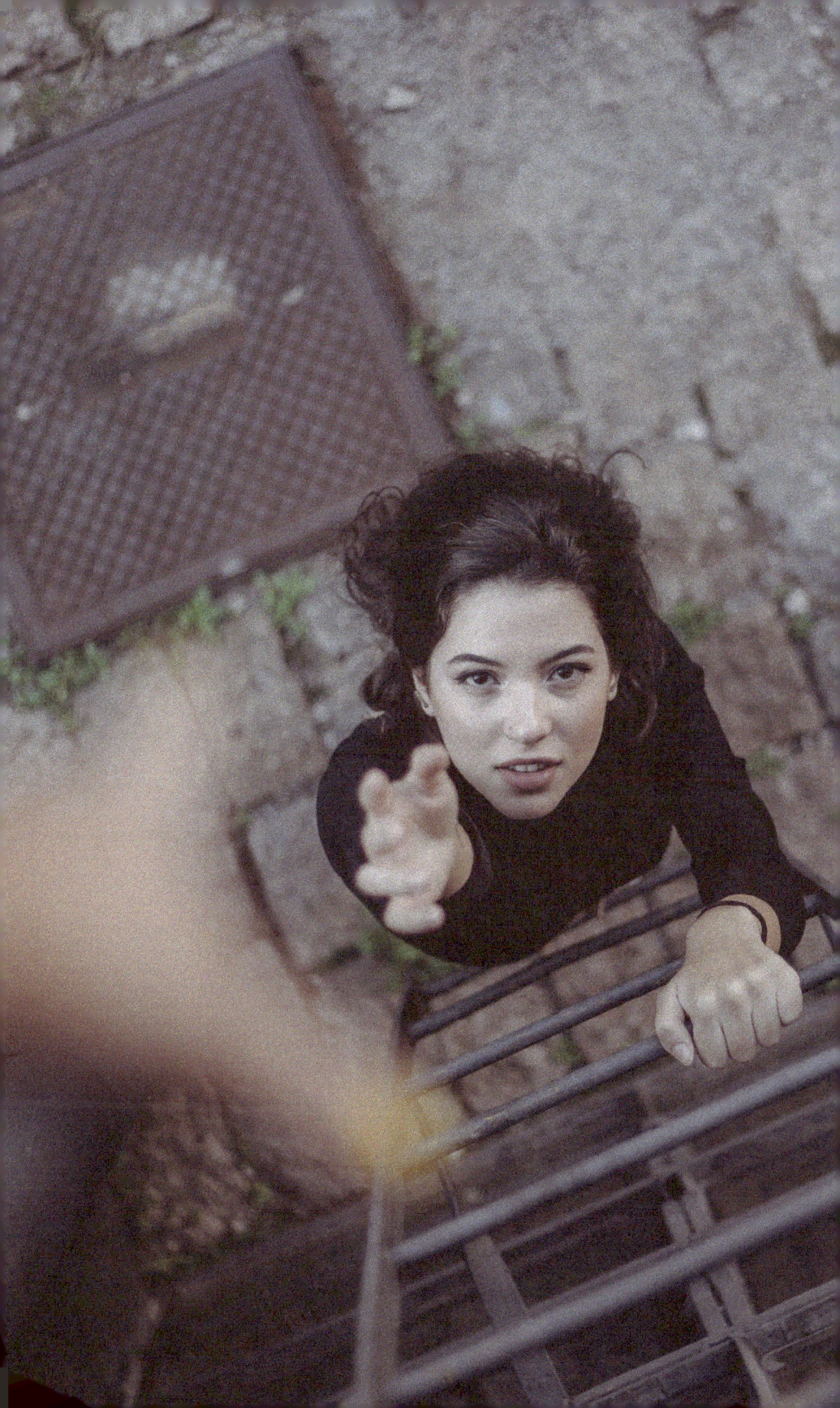

88

I want to give you back the gift of time this year. There are 24 hours in a day. Take a moment to reflect on how you'd like to spend your day today. Are there any interactions you need to have or want to have? Is there anything you absolutely must do? Anyone you truly need to have a conversation with? Let's talk about it.

89

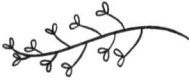

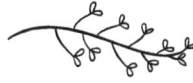

"The only courage you need is the courage to live your dreams" (Oprah Winfrey). I read this quote years ago and added it to my signature at work. You don't realize how brave you are to take steps to live the life you've set out for yourself. I remember back in college, my parents wanted me to be a doctor, lawyer, or nurse. I tried for two years, until I realized this wasn't the life I wanted for myself. I decided to switch my major for the fourth time and somehow ended up in tech. It's not always going to be easy to walk in the life you've dreamed up. I encourage you (and so does Oprah) to try it. What is it you've been waiting for? What adventure are you ready to embark on? Tell me about your journey!

....

....

....

....

....

....

....

....

....

....

....

....

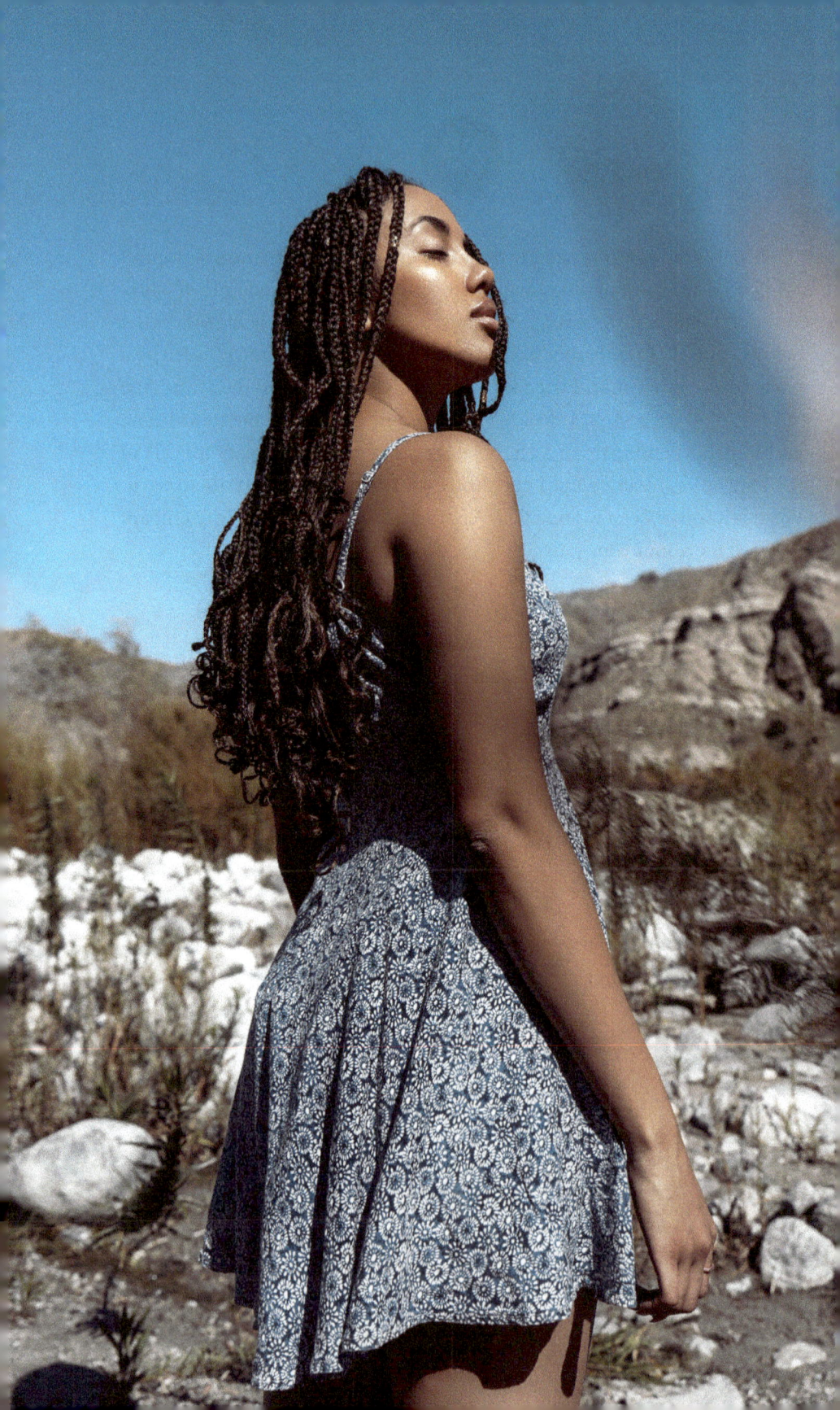

90

"Vision is what you see with your eyes closed. Sight is what you see with your eyes open" (Michael Todd). Take a look at your surroundings. What do you see? Now close your eyes, and what do you envision for your life?

....

....

....

....

....

....

....

....

....

....

....

....

....

....

....

91

You're an amazing person! You are on top of your game! You spread love, joy, and positivity! Self-encouragement. Positive speak. Words of affirmation. However you label it. You are your best cheerleader. Spend some time reflecting on just how awesome you are. Whatever you do, don't stop. Let the pen keep moving for at least five minutes. #selfcare #selflove #selfconfidence #selfcare

92

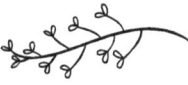

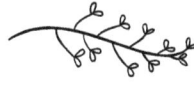

"Focus on things that are small enough to change, but big enough to matter! Choose to be happy! Don't focus on what's wrong. Find something positive in your life!" (Stephanie Henry). Count to 10 and write down 10 things in your life that are motivating you right now. If you can't think of 10, focus on what you have and just write. The idea is to keep the pen moving for at least ten minutes.

....

....

....

....

....

....

....

....

....

....

....

....

....

....

93

Bruce Lee said that the quest for truth is only better when you're meant to take action on what you find. Some of us are afraid to live in our truths. Some of us boldly live in our truths. For today's prompt, I want you to write about what your truth is. How have you come to this realization and how are you able to constantly be motivated by that inside you?

94

"Our stories are our power" (A'Lelia Bundles). Madam C.J. Walker's great-granddaughter, A'Lelia Bundles, shares with us that your story is your truth. It's your power, and it's yours to tell. How will you use your story to influence others?

95

"It starts with you! The world that comes to you, you choose how you see it!" (Daybreaker). What is life giving you right now? How are you welcoming these things?

....
....
....
....
....
....
....
....
....
....
....
....
....
....
....
....
....

96

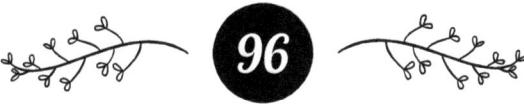

Joy is revolutionary! Happiness shouldn't be the goal. The goal is to be whole. Today, I want you to meditate on everything which makes you whole. Your career, your school, your family, friends, dog, cat. The goal is to be whole. What things/people make YOU whole?

97

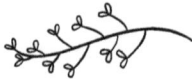

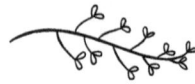

"The commitment to do well and to be well is a lifetime of choices that you make daily. The space to live in is not "I'll try" ... It's "I have decided." What will you commit today? To be well and maintain a sense of well-being you must commit to new habits and choose to practice them consistently. The results are in the choices. Write down 3-5 commitments for your well-being journey. It can be some of our mindful practices discussed in the education portion, it can be self-affirmation lists on a weekly basis. What's your commitment today?

....

....

....

....

....

....

....

....

....

....

....

....

....

....

98

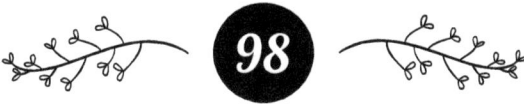

R.W.A.: Real Work Ahead. In today's prompt, we reflect on how the real work is ahead. If you're like me, sometimes when things don't go as planned, I say "Maybe it's a sign" or "I'll get the next one." Sometimes I even ponder on giving up. During my run today, I was reminded that the Real Work is Ahead. I saw a sign which said "Road Work Ahead" and thought to myself, if that's not the truth! 1. I need to continue running, as I was training for a marathon. 2. So many things in my life I've buried, or thought, "oh it's too late, I'm too old for that dream now. My time has passed." No! Taking these thoughts captive. I convinced myself instead that the Real Work is Ahead. Now is not the time to give up. The sign was so apropos in this situation. I needed to keep swimming, keep running, and just know if it was easy, then someone else would've already done it. My time is now. RWA. What real work do you have ahead?

....
....
....
....
....
....
....
....
....
....

99

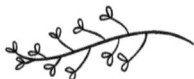

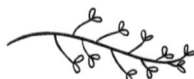

"The time will come when, with elation, you will greet yourself arriving at your own door, in your own mirror, and each will smile at the other's welcome, and say, sit here. Eat. You will love again the stranger who was your self" (Derek Walcott). That quote is from the poem, "Love after Love Exerts." I wanted to introduce toward the end of the book as a reminder which is; Your Life. Your Journey. Throughout this book, you've done the work to discover parts of yourself you may have never fully or deeply explored. There are now some key foundations which play a critical part in your growth and maturity as you navigate this huge world. The "Love after Love" poem allows you to come face-to-face with your old self while birthing your new self. Smile at this person. Love this person. They are your biggest critic, but also your #1 cheerleader, fan, and best friend. Self-love is the best love, because without self-love, it's impossible to render the same love to others. So love yourself, my friend. Understand who you truly are, and who it is you are becoming. Life is a marathon, not a sprint. Reflect on your old self in the mirror and write about this new self you see.

....

....

....

....

....

....

....

....

100

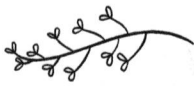

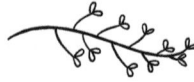

I got 99 prompts and this here mines! Create your last prompt. Full creative license here.

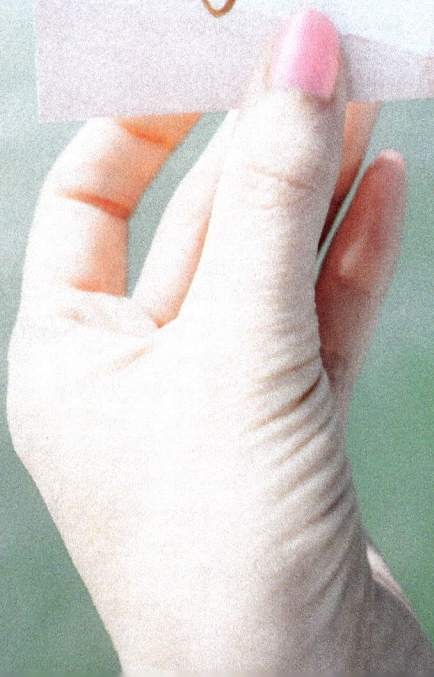

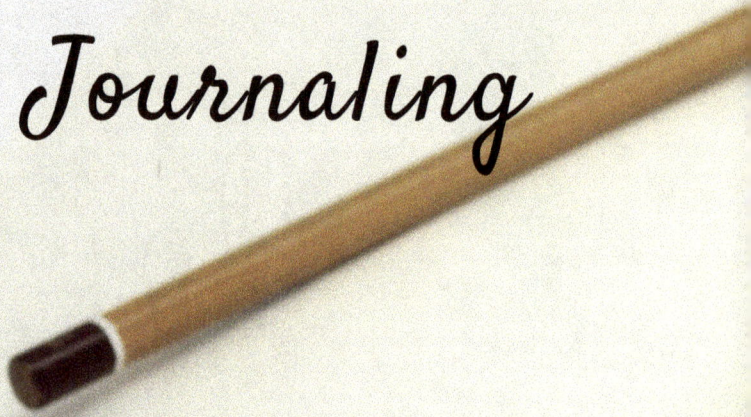

Journaling

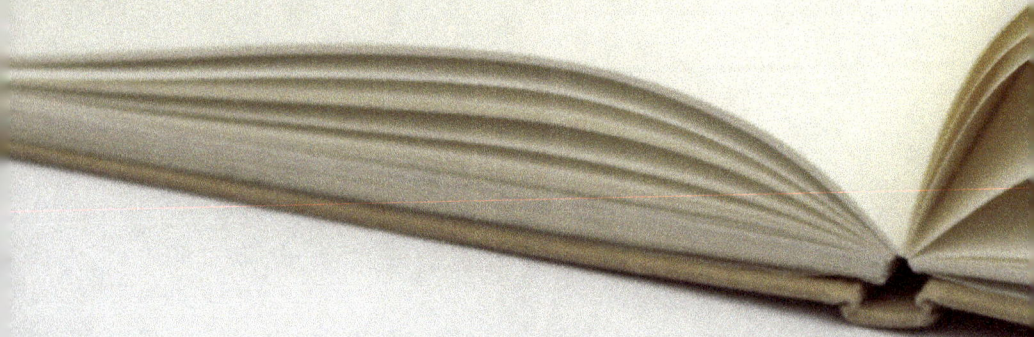

Here are a few additional pages for you to expand on prompts you've really enjoyed or take some additional time to reflect on the better version of you!

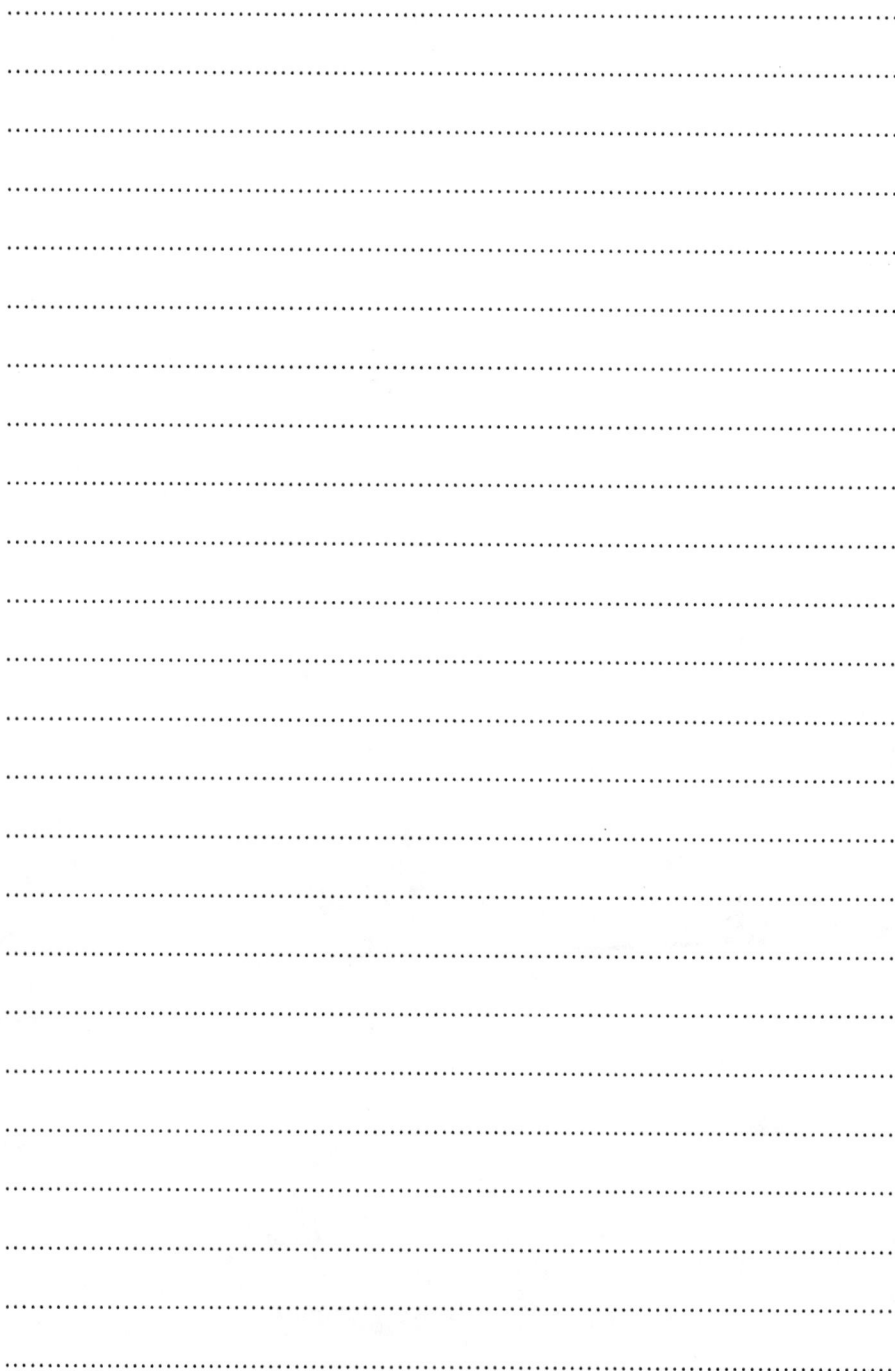

Notes

Prompt 1. "Mindful Nation UK Report." *The Mindfulness Initiative,* www.themindful-nessinitiative.org/mindful-nation-report.

Prompt 2. Oprah Vision Tour- attendee Full interview can be found here: https://www.youtube.com/watch?v=T_cCbsUKhwI

Prompt 3. Mental Health Foundation. 2020. *Mindfulness.* [online] Available at: <https://www.mentalhealth.org.uk/a-to-z/m/mindfulness> [Accessed 11 September 2020].

Prompt 7. Verywell Mind. 2020. *Know More. Live Brighter.* [online] Available at: <https://www.verywellmind.com/> [Accessed 11 September 2020].

Prompt 9. Nazish, N., 2020. *Why Sunlight Is Actually Good For You.* [online] Forbes. Available at: <https://www.forbes.com/sites/nomanazish/2018/02/28/why-sun-light-is-actually-good-for-you/#4a8bf2bf5cd9> [Accessed 11 September 2020].

Prompt 10. Killingsworth, M. and Gilbert, D., 2010. A Wandering Mind Is an Unhappy Mind. *Science,* 330(6006), pp.932-932.

Prompt 11. UniversalClass.com. 2020. *The 3 Basic Listening Models And How To Effectively Use Them.* [online] Available at: <https://www.universalclass.com/articles/business/listening-models.htm> [Accessed 11 September 2020].

Prompt 13. Seligman, M., 2008. Positive Health. *Applied Psychology,* 57(s1), pp.3-18.

Prompt 14. 2020. [online] Available at: <https://www.uvmhealth.org/coronavirus/staying-healthy/3-minute-anxiety-activity> [Accessed 11 September 2020].

Prompt 18. Strecher, V., 2017. *Life On Purpose.* [Place of publication not identified]: Harpercollins.

Prompt 23. APA. "Open Up! Writing About Trauma Reduces Stress, Aids Immunity." American Psychological Association. American Psychological Association, October 23, 2003. https://www.apa.org/research/action/writing

Prompt 26. BrainyQuote. 2020. *Jack Welch Quotes.* [online] Available at: <https://www.brainyquote.com/quotes/jack_welch_833427> [Accessed 11 September 2020].

Prompt 30. Facebook.com. 2020. *Wildbird.* [online] Available at: <https://www.facebook.com/mywildbird/photos/choosing-to-love-myself-is-where-i-found-my-power-alex-elle-alex_elle-because-th/2804743463086566/> [Accessed 11 September 2020].

Prompt 31. Inspiring Quotes. 2020. *Top 30 Quotes Of TINA TURNER Famous Quotes And Sayings | Inspringquotes.Us.* [online] Available at: <https://www.inspiringquotes.us/author/1801-tina-turner> [Accessed 11 September 2020].

Prompt 34. Oprah Vision Tour- attendee Full interview can be found here. https://www.youtube.com/watch?v=T_cCbsUKhwI

Prompt 37. Day, D., 1956. *Que Sera, Sera (Whatever Will Be, Will Be).*

Prompt 41. Wiseoldsayings.com. 2020. *Sarah Ban Breathnach Quotes And Sayings | Wise Old Sayings.* [online] Available at: <https://www.wiseoldsayings.com/authors/sarah-ban-breathnach--quotes/> [Accessed 11 September 2020].

Prompt 42. A quote from Unashamed. (n.d.). Retrieved from https://www.goodreads.com/quotes/8959968-if-you-live-for-people-s-acceptance-you-ll-die-from-their

Prompt 46. Goodreads.com. 2020. *A Quote By Kobe Bryant.* [online] Available at: <https://www.goodreads.com/quotes/7691569-i-have-self-doubt-i-have-insecurity-i-have-fear-of> [Accessed 11 September 2020].

Prompt 47. A quote by Maya Angelou. (n.d.). Www.Goodreads.Com. Retrieved September 11, 2020, from, https://www.goodreads.com/quotes/700564-if-you-are-always-trying-to-be-normal-you-will

Prompt 48. thompson, april. (2018). Darkness cannot drive out darkness; only LIGHT can do that... Martin Luther King Jr. In *YouTube.* https://www.youtube.com/watch?v=Fyg2f9at0FI

Prompt 49. SuperSoul on Facebook Watch. (n.d.). Www.Facebook.Com. Retrieved September 11, 2020, from https://www.facebook.com/watch/?v=1525422300838618

Prompt 54. Oprah Vision Tour- attendee Full interview can be found here: https://www.youtube.com/watch?v=T_cCbsUKhwI

Prompt 59. Oprah Vision Tour- attendee Full interview can be found here: https://www.youtube.com/watch?v=T_cCbsUKhwI

Prompt 61. Tennyson, A. T. (1850). *In memoriam.* London: E. Moxon.

Prompt 70. "Never be limited by other people's imaginations" (Dr. Mae Jemison) Speech

Prompt 72. Theodore Roosevelt Quote: "Comparison is the thief of joy". (2020). Retrieved 11 September 2020, from, https://quotefancy.com/quote/33048/Theodore-Roosevelt-Comparison-is-the-thief-of-joy

Prompt 75. Williamson, M., Fear, O., & Williamson, M. (2020). Our Deepest Fear Poem by Marianne Williamson - Poem Hunter. Retrieved 11 September 2020, from https://www.poemhunter.com/poem/our-deepest-fear-5/

Prompt 81. Martin Seligman on Psychology. (2020). Retrieved 11 September 2020, from https://www.pursuit-of-happiness.org/history-of-happiness/martin-seligman-psychology/

Prompt 88. Nic Hepton. Well-Being Speech

Prompt 89. A quote by Oprah Winfrey. (2020). Retrieved 11 September 2020, from, https://www.goodreads.com/quotes/554552-you-ve-got-to-follow-your-passion-you-ve-got-to-figure

Prompt 90. "Vision is what you see with your eyes closed. Sight is what you see with your eyes open" (Michael Todd) Transformation Church 2020

Prompt 92. "Focus on things that are small enough to change, but big enough to matter! Choose to be happy! Don't focus on what's wrong. Find something positive in your life!" (Stephanie Henry) Family Relative

Prompt 93. Best Bruce Lee Quotes. (2020). Retrieved 11 September 2020, from https://sourcesofinsight.com/bruce-lee-quotes/#:~:text=Top%2010%20Bruce%20Lee%20Quotes

Prompt 94. A'Lelia Bundles | Author, Journalist, Truth Seeker. (2020). Retrieved 11 September 2020, from https://aleliabundles.com/

Prompt 95. "It starts with you! The world that comes to you, you choose how you see it!" (Daybreaker) Oprah's Vision 2020 Tour

Prompt 97. Oprah Makes the Commitment. (2020). Retrieved 11 September 2020, from https://www.oprah.com/health/making-the-commitment/all

Prompt 99. Love after love - Derek Walcott | Mindfulness Association. (2020). Retrieved 11 September 2020, from https://www.mindfulnessassociation.net/words-of-wonder/love-after-love-derek-walcott/